THE FOOD
HOSPI+AL

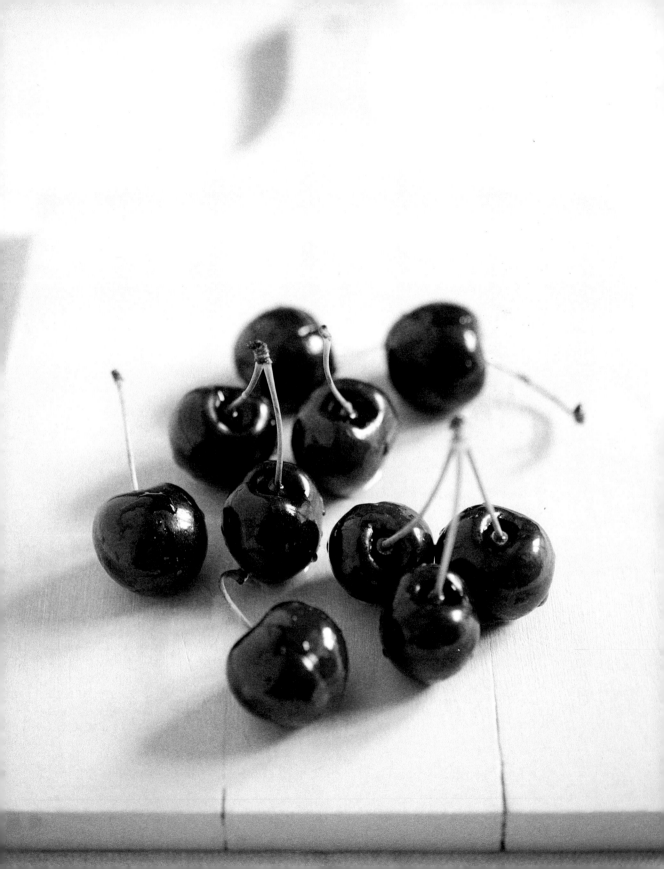

THE FOOD HOSPITAL

SIMPLE, DELICIOUS RECIPES FOR A HEALTHY LIFE

DR GIO MILETTO,
LUCY JONES, DR SHAW SOMERS

photography by Susan Bell

MICHAEL JOSEPH
an imprint of
Penguin Books

MICHAEL JOSEPH

Published by the Penguin Group

Penguin Books Ltd, 80 Strand, London WC2R 0RL, England

Penguin Group (USA) Inc., 375 Hudson Street, New York, New York 10014, USA

Penguin Group (Canada), 90 Eglinton Avenue East, Suite 700, Toronto, Ontario, Canada M4P 2YR
(a division of Pearson Penguin Canada Inc.)

Penguin Ireland, 25 St Stephen's Green, Dublin 2, Ireland
(a division of Penguin Books Ltd)

Penguin Group (Australia), 250 Camberwell Road, Camberwell, Victoria 3124, Australia (a division of Pearson Australia Group Pty Ltd)

Penguin Books India Pvt Ltd, 11 Community Centre, Panchsheel Park, New Delhi – 110 017, India

Penguin Group (NZ), 67 Apollo Drive, Rosedale, Auckland 0632, New Zealand (a division of Pearson New Zealand Ltd)

Penguin Books (South Africa) (Pty) Ltd, 24 Sturdee Avenue, Rosebank, Johannesburg 2196, South Africa

Penguin Books Ltd, Registered Offices: 80 Strand, London WC2R 0RL England

www.penguin.com

First published 2011

5

Copyright © Betty tv ltd 2011

Photography copyright © Susan Bell, 2011

The moral right of the authors has been asserted

Set in Nimbus Sans Novus T, Rockwell Std and Sevigne

Printed and bound by Firmengruppe APPL, aprinta druck, Wemding, Germany

A CIP catalogue record for this book is available from the British Library

978-0-718-15859-0

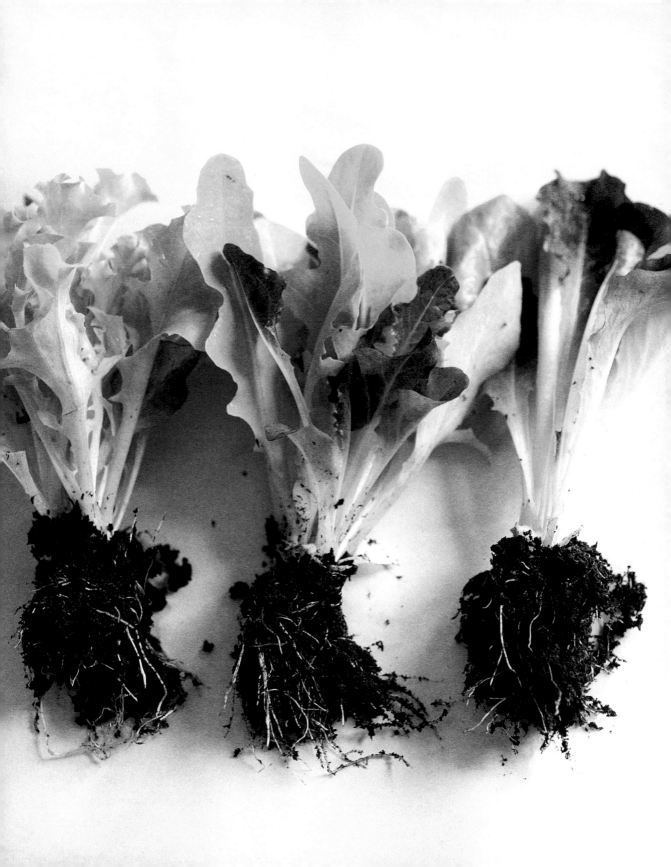

CONTENTS

EAT YOURSELF BETTER 170

WHEN THINGS GET SERIOUS 214

INTRODUCTION

Fifty years ago, health was seen as the absence of disease. If you didn't have smallpox or diabetes or rheumatoid arthritis, you could count yourself lucky, even if you had loads of niggling minor health problems. Sanitation improved in the late 1950s and early 1960s: you got the builders to bring the outside lavvy inside and paid attention to the rudimentary government advice on washing your hands before preparing food. When your eyesight got blurry, you picked up a pair of NHS specs, and when your teeth fell out, you had a set of dentures fitted – but that was about the extent of the responsibility you took for your own health.

In the twenty-first century, as the result of decades of research being broadcast in the media, we understand a lot more about how our health is affected by the world we live in. We know that asbestos is an environmental hazard, and that the sun's UV rays can cause skin cancer, and at last the message on smoking has got through. No smoker in 2011 can claim they didn't realize it was bad for them!

On top of that, we are becoming better educated about nutrition, and the ways in which the food we put in our mouths affect our general health and life expectancy. Fifty years ago, we might have taken a packed lunch to work consisting of Spam sandwiches on white bread, and some people might even have added a sprinkling of table salt. Nowadays, most of us understand that eating is not just about putting fuel in the tank to keep us going, as if we were some kind of machine. There's a much more subtle relationship between food and the human body. Particular genes in our DNA may be turned on or off in response to nutrition and the environment. Our hormones and blood pressure are affected by what we eat. We get pleasure from eating good food, and that is important for our wellbeing in itself.

By choosing our foods carefully, we can have a lot more control than we ever have over how well we age, how we resist illnesses, and the number of years we are able to live an active life. We at The Food Hospital have compiled some of the latest research on how you can use food to prevent and alleviate illness, and we'd like to share it with you.

FORGET ABOUT THE MAGIC PILL

A downside of all the attention-grabbing headlines about nutrition in magazines and newspapers is that we have come to expect magic solutions to all our problems: a seven-day detox diet, a handful of goji berries, or a multivitamin pill grabbed on the run when we haven't had time to eat a proper meal. We look for a quick fix that will undo the effects of an unhealthy lifestyle over many years, a diet secret that will mean we effortlessly reach our ideal weight and a supplement to prevent us ever getting cancer. Well, we're afraid none of these exist. Sorry!

There are no shortcuts when it comes to healthy eating. You can't undo damage done over a year with a week of detoxing, and modern dietitians will always advise you to eat a balanced diet with a wide variety of foods, rather than gulping down vitamin and mineral supplements to make up deficiencies. A little knowledge can be a dangerous thing because someone might swallow a supplement they've read about to address one problem, and find that it is affecting their absorption of other nutrients, causing whole new problems. As just one example, taking an iron supplement can impair your absorption of calcium and zinc, which are both just as necessary for good health.

No micronutrient works in isolation. They're all part of an intricate network of mechanisms for absorption, transport and metabolism. The great thing is that fresh, whole foods often contain a combination of essential vitamins and minerals along with the micronutrients necessary for their absorption – a kind of all-in-one solution. The more types of food you eat, the more likely it is that you are getting everything you need. You're probably familiar with the advice to eat five portions of fruit and veg a day – but if you only eat peas and bananas, you'll be missing out on a lot of essential nutrients. If you manage to eat thirty different fruits and vegetables in a week, you'll have a much better chance of covering all the bases.

The truth is that nutrition is a relatively new science and we don't understand everything about how the human body uses food. We're just beginning to realize some things, but what we do know is exciting, in that it can already help us to take more control over our health and wellbeing than we've ever had before.

THE EATWELL PLATE

Dietitians often base their advice for healthy eating around something called the Eatwell Plate and suggest that you try to make your own plate look like it at every meal. Here's how it works.

A third of your plate should be covered with starchy carbohydrates, such as potatoes, pasta, rice, noodles, couscous or even a slice of bread. That's right – carbs! Those who follow 'low-carb' and 'no-carb' diets are missing out on a range of important nutrients, including the B vitamins that are required for the health of your nervous system. Choose wholegrain whenever possible for the fibre it contains, and because when the grain is processed to make white flour products, most of the goodness is lost.

A third of your plate should be covered with fruits and vegetables of different colours. We get different nutrients from different-coloured plant foods, as you'll see from pages 11–13. In particular, we get a range of essential vitamins, minerals and antioxidants, which help to protect our cells from damage by molecules known as free radicals – these are created during the breakdown of foods or after exposure to cigarette smoke or radiation. Free radicals play a role in the development of cancer and heart disease, so it's important to get enough antioxidants in our diets to protect us.

Part of the remaining third will be for proteins – that's lean meat, poultry, fish, eggs and alternative proteins for vegetarians, such as tofu, beans and pulses, nuts and seeds. If you're a vegan or a non-dairy-eating vegetarian, you need to eat a good range of proteins to ensure you get sufficient amino acids, which form the building blocks of the body. Fortified cereals and soya or rice milk can help vegans to get the all-important vitamin B12 they need.

Another part of the Eatwell Plate is for dairy products – milk, cheese, butter and yoghurt. We should aim for three portions of dairy per day to get the calcium we need – but note that a 'portion' is just a 25g piece of cheese (the size of a matchbox), a small 150g pot of low-fat yoghurt or a 250ml glass of milk, so don't go mad.

A small sliver of your plate can be for foods and drinks that are high in fat or sugar, because some are necessary to add flavour. There's more about fat on page 16.

That's the way the proportions should work. If you look at a deep-pan four-cheese pizza, or a burger and chips 'meal', you can see that they don't fit the pattern at all. Try to adapt your meals to look like the Eatwell Plate, and you are well on the way to having a healthy diet. There are a couple more pieces of general advice you should take on board, and they concern carbohydrates and fats. See pages 14–16.

Brightly coloured fruits and vegetables are rich in a wide variety of antioxidants that have a host of health benefits. The body produces its own antioxidants, but some people can become deficient. Aim to eat a rainbow of foods every day to ensure that you are getting everything you need for optimum health and wellbeing.

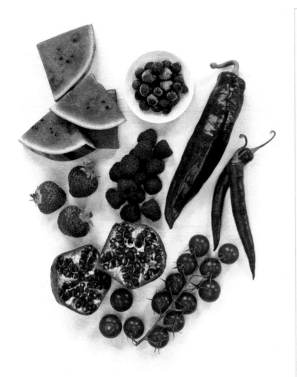

RED AND PINK

Almost all red fruit and vegetables contain lycopene, which reduces the risk of prostate cancer, and promotes colon health. Berries are rich in ellagic acid, which supports the immune system, and have antiviral and antibacterial qualities; they also contain anthocyanins, which can help slow down the degenerative processes of ageing, providing protection against a number of cancers and cardiovascular disease, as well as showing antiviral and antibacterial properties.

YELLOW AND ORANGE

The main antioxidants found in orange fruits and vegetables are carotenoids (which are also found in leafy green vegetables); these are a precursor to vitamin A, which is essential for healthy skin, eyes and mucous membranes (which line the urinary, digestive and respiratory tracts). Diets rich in beta-carotene (which gives these foods their orange colour) have been linked with a reduced risk of certain cancers and heart disease and play a role in immunity, bone health and age-related dementia.

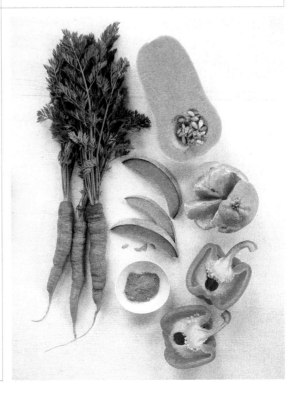

GREEN

Lutein, found in all dark green plant foods (as well as yellow and orange fruits and vegetables), is important for healthy vision, and helps to prevent degeneration of the eyes, as well as the development of cataracts. Dark, leafy green vegetables are rich in carotenoids (see Yellow and Orange), as well as zeaxanthin, which may help to reduce the risk of certain types of cancer, such as breast and lung cancer, and may contribute to the prevention of heart disease and stroke. They also contain quercetin (see White), which can act as an anti-inflammatory.

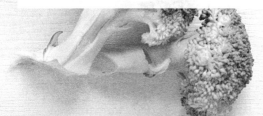

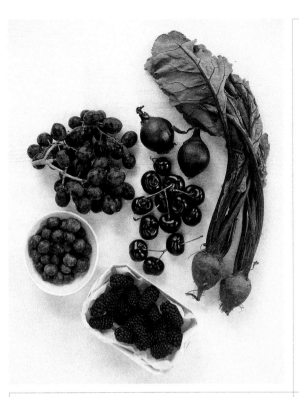

PURPLE AND BLUE

The flavonoids found in red grapes (known as resveratrol) promote a healthy heart and circulatory system, while blueberries and blackberries contain ellagic acid (see Red and Pink) and catechins, which can help to prevent cancer. Rich in anthocyanins, purple and blue foods can also reduce the risk of cancer, improve the health of your urinary tract and encourage healthy memory and ageing. Blueberries, in particular, have been proven to reduce mental decline (including Alzheimer's) and protect against inflammation.

WHITE

Onions and garlic contain protective phytonutrients (plant nutrients) that can reduce the risk of cancer; these include quercetin and allicin, which are known to kill harmful bacteria and protect the capillaries. Mushrooms are high in antioxidant polyphenols, which are known to reduce the risk of heart disease, while cauliflower contains compounds such as glucosinolates and thiocyanates that can protect against heart disease, cancer, digestive disorders and obesity. Oats and flaxseed contain lignan, which is known to lower cholesterol, prevent kidney disease and balance hormones (i.e. during menopause), while nuts and seeds contain anti-inflammatory compounds.

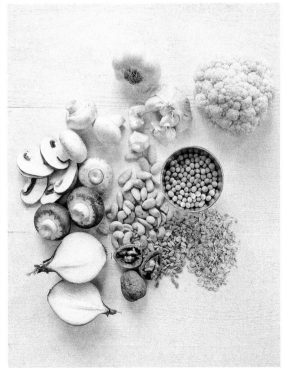

EAT LOW-GL FOODS

There's a tool called the Glycaemic Index that dietitians recommend you use when planning your meals. It's a ranking of carbohydrate foods based on their effects on our blood sugar levels and was originally developed for diabetics. Glycaemic Load (GL) takes into account the Glycaemic Index rating of a food as well as the portion size to give the most accurate way of predicting how foods affect our blood sugar. Eating foods that are low on the GL scale can improve the health of all of us. Here's how it works.

Foods that are absorbed into the bloodstream slowly have a low GL rating, while those that are absorbed quickly have a high rating. By choosing mainly low-GL foods, you prevent blood sugar peaks and troughs that can cause energy dips, hunger and light-headedness, as well as mood swings and irritability. Keeping your blood sugar stable is also good for weight control and, as you'll see in the rest of the book, keeping your weight at a healthy level is one of the most important things you can do for your overall health. It also helps to reduce insulin reisistance, a known issue in a

Low GL	Medium GL	High GL
• 1 slice of wholemeal bread	• 2 tablespoons honey	• A slice of French bread or a bagel
• A bowl of porridge	• A serving of instant oatmeal	• An average serving of cornflakes, sugary cereals or cereal containing dried fruit
• A small bowl of popcorn	• A medium croissant with butter	
• A glass of tomato juice	• A slice of cake	• A portion of white rice or couscous
• A serving of cooked lentils, soya or kidney beans	• A glass of apple juice	• 2 teaspoons sugar
	• A cup of hot chocolate	• A medium blueberry muffin
• A large carrot or a serving of peas, tomato, broccoli, cabbage, cauliflower, mushroom, spinach – most vegetables	• A serving of chickpeas of baked beans	• A medium baked potato
	• A portion of pasta al dente	• A portion of sweetcorn or corn on the cob
	• A portion of brown rice	
• An average portion of melon, papaya, kiwi, orange, grapes, strawberries, apple, pear, peach, plum – most fruit	• A portion of mashed or boiled potato	• A handful of dried fruits, such as raisins, dried apricots, prunes, dates
	• An average serving of sweet potato or yam	• A can of fizzy drink, such as cola or orangeade
• A handful of nuts and seeds	• An average portion of fresh pineapple, banana, mango or fruits canned in syrup	
• A glass of milk, small pot of yoghurt or a scoop of ice cream		

variety of health conditions. Opposite, you'll find a list of low- and high-GL foods. If in doubt, apply some general rules:

- **If a food tastes sweet,** it is probably high-GL.

- **If it's made from refined white flour,** it will have a higher GL rating than its wholegrain equivalent.

- **Fibre slows the absorption of carbs,** so a whole apple will have a lower GL than a glass of apple juice.

- **Proteins and fats slow down the digestion of carbs,** so they can reduce the effect of a higher-GL food on your blood. That's why it's better to have a boiled egg with your toast, rather than jam or marmalade.

- **Get into the habit of eating the low-GL way and you will reap the benefits** in terms of lessened risk of serious disease and more stable energy levels.

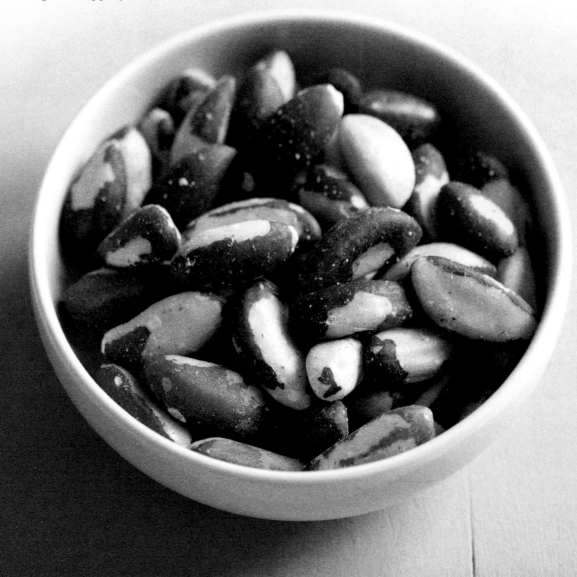

CHOOSE YOUR FATS WISELY

There are three main types of fat – saturated, monounsaturated and polyunsaturated – and they all have different roles in the body. You've probably heard saturated fats being vilified left, right and centre, but that's only because we eat too many of them (in red meat, butter, cheese, burgers, sausages – basically, animal fats are saturated, as are coconut and palm oils). A certain amount of saturated fat is needed to manufacture cell walls and for other metabolic purposes in the body, but when we eat too much our cholesterol levels rise and our arteries get clogged up, leading to heart disease and strokes.

Eating the right kinds of fat can help to protect you from heart and circulatory problems. Monounsaturated fats, found in olive, groundnut and rapeseed oils and spreads, and in nuts, olives and avocados, are particularly good for heart health. Polyunsaturated fats help us to burn the energy from food and contain three very important groups of fat: the omega 3, omega 6 and omega 9 fats. Omega 3s are found in oily fish – salmon, mackerel, trout, sardines and herring – as well as in flaxseed, walnuts and pumpkin seeds. They help to prevent your arteries from getting clogged up and lower your blood pressure, and that's why dietitians recommend that we eat at least one serving of oily fish a week. Omega 6 fats are found in pumpkin, sunflower, sesame, corn and soya oil, as well as nuts and seeds, and they also have beneficial effects on the heart and circulation when eaten in moderation. Omega 9 oils reduce insulin resistance (which helps to prevent obesity and diabetes), encourage immunity, reduce the risk of hardening of the arteries, and lower cholesterol levels. They are found in olives, olive oil, avocados, almonds, sesame seeds, pecans, peanuts, cashews and hazelnuts. The best advice is to simplify your store cupboard so that it contains olive oil for dressing salads and rapeseed oil for cooking.

There's another group of fats that have got a bad name and that's transfats, aka hydrogenated fats. These are used in shop-bought pies, pastries and cakes, particularly, and are linked to high cholesterol levels and increased risk of heart disease and cancer. Read the labels on any foods you haven't cooked from fresh and try to give these fats a wide berth.

So there are good fats and bad fats when it comes to health – but they are all fattening. A tablespoon of healthy olive oil and a tablespoon of unhealthy lard both have 135 calories. It's worth remembering as you glug oil into your wok for a stir-fry or dribble dressing over your salad …

FOOD AS MEDICINE

We've outlined the basic principles for healthy eating using the Eatwell Plate, but in this book we're going to go further and look at ways you can use food to prevent and treat some common illnesses and health conditions. Food affects our immunity to viruses, it affects our hormone balance, and it affects the composition of our blood and the nutrients and energy available to our cells, so it stands to reason that some foods will help when a particular body system isn't working efficiently, while other foods might exacerbate the condition.

Using food as medicine is a continually developing science. Every week, the results of new studies are announced, which clarify, develop and sometimes even contradict the previously received wisdom. It's an exciting area of healthcare, but because the body of evidence about what works and what doesn't is still emerging, many of the recommendations have yet to be incorporated into the mainstream. That's why it's essential that you don't make any dramatic changes to your diet based on advise you read in this book, or in articles you read in the newspapers, without checking with a health professional first. Most of the nutritional recommendations we offer here are based on published studies, but we have also included anecdotal evidence where we feel it might be of interest, or worth a discussion. For example, we all know people who have excluded wheat from their diet and realized they feel much better for it. They don't have coeliac disease, in which there is an immune reaction to a protein found in wheat (see page 34), but they find that certain symptoms, such as tiredness or bloating, are relieved when they avoid it. We can't back this up with hard scientific evidence but it seems that some people benefit from excluding certain foods from their diet and, so long as they don't cut out a whole food group (such as all carbohydrates), they aren't doing any harm.

In this book, we might recommend that you exclude a few common 'trigger foods' from your diet to see if the symptoms of a health problem are relieved. This is called an 'exclusion diet'. You should exclude the food in question for around four weeks, while keeping an eye on your symptoms to see if they clear up. If there is no change after four weeks, you might as well reintroduce the food. Even if your symptoms improve during the exclusion period, you should start eating the food in question again after four weeks to see if they get worse once more, because that will give you further evidence that the food was responsible. Exclusion diets should never be tried on children without medical supervision.

Some conditions, such as eczema and asthma, may have a number of different triggers. In this case, you should exclude trigger foods one at a time, while keeping a food and symptom diary to see if you can work out a pattern that would indicate that a particular food might be the culprit. It's OK to exclude single foods, such as citrus fruits or tomatoes, but don't ever exclude a whole group, such as dairy, without the support of a qualified dietitian, because you could find

yourself becoming deficient in other essential nutrients. Note that some people may struggle to find any triggers at all; it's not a foregone conclusion by any means.

An intolerance to a particular foodstuff is quite different from a food allergy. In an allergy, the immune system over-reacts to the presence of a trigger substance in a way that can be life-threatening. In peanut allergy, for instance, when even a trace of a protein found in peanuts is consumed, the immune system can go into overdrive and the patient can experience vomiting, diarrhoea, breathing difficulties, hives, a swelling of the face, lips and tongue, acute abdominal pain – a collection of symptoms known as anaphylactic shock – which can cause death. Symptoms of an allergy are experienced either immediately after or sometimes several hours after the substance has been eaten, whereas if you have an intolerance to a foodstuff, the symptoms may build up gradually over a period of weeks, months or years. If you suspect you have a food allergy, you should speak to your doctor and ask to be referred to an allergy specialist.

The nutritional advice related to health conditions in this book can be used if you already have a health condition you want to treat, or if you have a genetic predisposition to a particular disease (in other words, if you have a strong family history) and want to minimize your chances of succumbing to it. We don't want to encourage self-diagnosis and treatment of serious ailments, which you should always discuss with your doctor. But educating yourself about your own health, and eating a varied diet with all the nutrients required for your body to function at its optimal levels, has got to be a giant evolutionary step forward from those Spam-sandwich-eating folk back in 1961.

'Aim to eat a rainbow of foods every day to ensure you are getting everything you need for optimum health and wellbeing.'

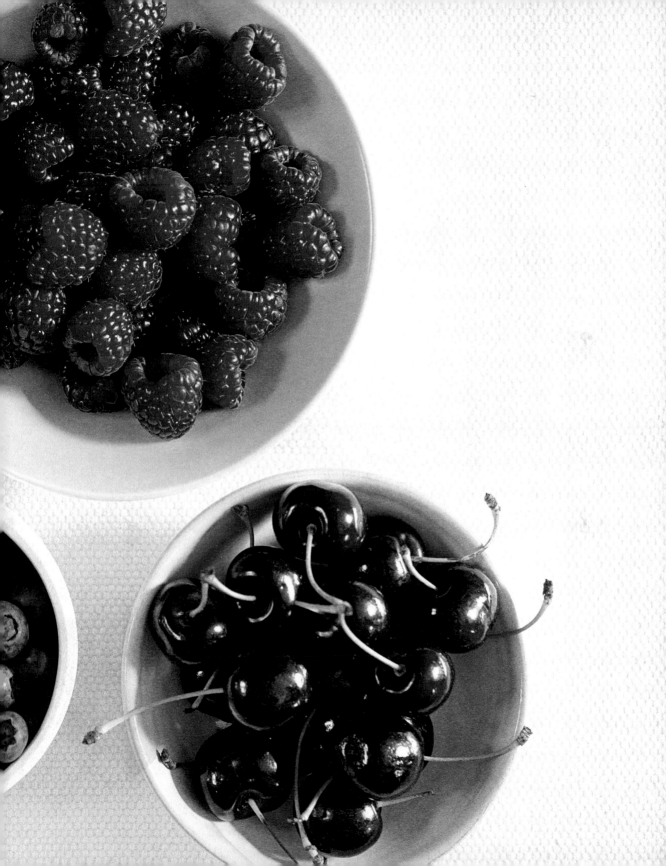

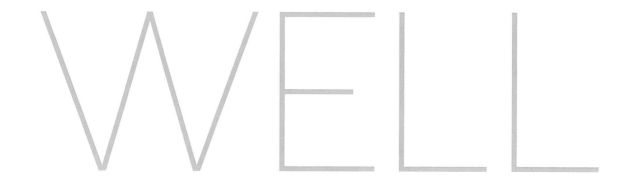

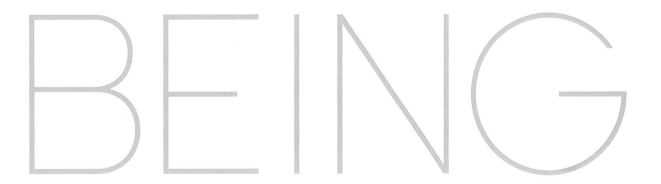

WELLBEING QUIZ

How much do you think you understand about looking after your own health? It can sometimes feel as if the more you know, the more confusing it gets, because one day the newspapers might report the results of a particular research study and the following week or month there will be another trial claiming the opposite. For example, should you take an aspirin a day to prevent heart disease? Should women eat lots of soya foods? The answers are not straightforward but are full of qualifications (see page 228 and chapter four for some thoughts on these topics).

However, there are some things that we know for sure are good for us, and likely to promote good health – and some things that are so bad they are likely to shorten our lives. Perhaps you are aware of them already – but are you implementing them in your life or do you always find some excuse (such as lack of time) for not doing what you know you should? On the following pages you will find a quiz that will test how well you are looking after yourself. Note down your answers, then check your score on page 24.

THE QUIZ

For each question, note all the answers that you feel apply to you.

1. I smoke . . .

A. only when I'm awake ☐

B. passively, when I'm around other people who are smoking ☐

C. socially (in other words, when I'm drunk) ☐

D. never have, never will ☐

E. I used to but managed to quit ☐

F. only non-tobacco products/cigars/hookahs. ☐

2. I eat . . .

A. lots of fresh fruit and veg every day ☐

B. a smoothie whenever I feel run-down ☐

C. the odd orange or apple for lunch ☐

D. a daily multivitamin because I don't like fruit and veg ☐

E. microwave chicken korma for its vegetable content ☐

F. usually on the run, between meetings. ☐

3. As far as colds and flu go . . .

A. I get the flu vaccine every year ☐

B. I use alternative remedies to prevent illness as I don't trust vaccines ☐

C. I believe I have a strong immunity so don't get vaccines ☐

D. I probably catch a cold once or twice a year, if that ☐

E. I have a cold every other week and tend to get mouth ulcers a lot ☐

F. I'm too exhausted to catch a cold. ☐

4. I drink alcohol . . .

A. never ☐

B. far more than I should but I seem to be getting away with it ☐

C. in the morning, at lunch, after work, and throughout the evenings; I need it to get through the day ☐

D. I'll sometimes have a glass of wine with my evening meal ☐

E. a few times a week, but I rarely get drunk ☐

F. with my mates at the weekends, because we can sleep off the hangover on Sundays. ☐

5. Preparing food is . . .

A. so last century and not necessary any more thanks to ready meals and vitamin supplements ☐

B. opening a jar, maybe boiling something, an occasional roast ☐

C. choosing whether to go with the large fries or the four-cheese pizza ☐

D. too much pressure; I'm not a celebrity chef ☐

E. enjoyable, regular and usually with other people ☐

F. enjoyable, regular and usually on my own. ☐

6. Exercise is . . .

A. something I admire other people for doing ☐

B. one of those things I just don't enjoy ☐

C. incorporated into my day by cycling to work ☐

D. so necessary to me that I get annoyed that the gym is closed at 3am ☐

E. a weekend activity ☐

F. something that gets my heart rate up most days of the week for more than half an hour at a time. ☐

7. As far as my weight goes . . .

A. I want to lose a few pounds ☐

B. I want to gain a few pounds ☐

C. I never weigh myself because I'm scared of what the scales might say ☐

D. I know I'm overweight but it's because I have a slow metabolism ☐

E. I'm happy as I am ☐

F. I'm never happy with it. ☐

8. Sunshine is . . .

A. to be worshipped ☐

B. best experienced in a tanning salon ☐

C. something I enjoy, while wearing sunscreen ☐

D. something I don't have to worry about because I have dark skin ☐

E. to be avoided at all costs ☐

F. a type of cocktail they serve in my local bar. ☐

9. Visiting the doctor . . .

A. gets me a regular cervical smear test (women) ☐

B. reminds me to book a mammogram (women) ☐

C. is a wonderful opportunity for a rectal exam (men) ☐

D. means someone called an ambulance for me ☐

E. is a nightmare; I know my blood pressure will be high, so I don't go ☐

F. is what happens when I'm sick, not when I feel fine. ☐

10. When it comes to salt . . .

A. I add it to crisps to get that extra bite ☐

B. food tastes bland if I don't add more of it ☐

C. I check the salt content on labels but it's hard to know what they mean ☐

D. I avoid fast food because of the salt (and saturated fat) content ☐

E. I make sure to also add pepper ☐

F. I know how much I'm getting and where it comes from in my diet. ☐

SCORING

If you scored between 0 and 44 . . .

Your diet and lifestyle need a serious make-over. Keep reading because it's never too late to make yourself healthier.

If you scored between 44 and 90 . . .

You're not doing too badly but a little fine-tuning here and there could make a big difference to your long-term health prospects.

If you scored over 90 . . .

You're doing a great job at maintaining yourself and preventing health problems.

	A	B	C	D	E	F
1	0	2	1	10	9	0
2	10	7	6	5	2	3
3	8	2	2	8	0	0
4	10	0	0	6	6	2
5	1	3	0	2	8	8
6	3	2	8	1	5	10
7	0	0	0	0	0	0
8	2	0	8	8	4	0
9	5	5	10	0	2	2
10	0	0	4	5	0	10

Why did we score questions the way we did? Read on:

SMOKING

You can drink in moderation without it being harmful, but any smoking at all is dangerous, whether it is passive smoking, a cigar at Christmas or an occasional cigarette at parties. See pages 134–5 for more information about the harm smoking does to virtually every system in the body – including some startling facts you may not have been aware of. You *know* it's not good for you. Maybe you smoke because you think it helps you to deal with stress, or keeps your weight down, or cheers you up; but in fact you are kidding yourself, as any effects are temporary. See your doctor for help to quit if you need it. It's not always easy but if you are a smoker it is the single most important thing you can do to prevent serious health problems in the future, and to stop yourself dying prematurely.

FRESH VEGETABLES AND FRUIT

Fruit and veg are packed with nutrients that reduce your risk of serious health problems. Taking a multivitamin doesn't begin to make up for the lack of a range of multi-coloured fruits and veggies in your diet, and smoothies have fewer nutrients than whole fruits. If you've convinced yourself that you don't like fruit and veg, persevere until you re-educate your taste buds. Finely chop veggies into a casserole so you can barely detect them but are still getting the nutrients. Try a chopped pear on top of your breakfast cereal or a tomato salad on the side at lunchtime. If you're not used to preparing fresh fruit and veg, try some of the delicious and easy-to-follow recipes in this book.

COLDS AND FLU

Colds and flu are caused by viruses. While flu can be fatal – and is every year – colds are less severe. But if you have an unhealthy lifestyle and are under stress, or if you are over the age of fifty, you may have a weakened immune system and be more likely to get these kinds of infections. Despite some scare stories claiming vaccines (such as MMR) are dangerous to the population, there is no evidence to support this. The vaccine programme for smallpox has now eradicated the disease worldwide, and the flu vaccine can prevent fatalities. The fact is, even if you choose not to be vaccinated, you are protected by the majority of people who have, because there is less of the illness spreading. Vaccines teach your immune system how to fight infections without the risk of getting the disease, and are well worth having.

ALCOHOL

One unit of alcohol a day – any kind – may slightly reduce your risk of heart disease (particularly for men). However, the health benefits stop after that. No doubt, good beers and wines are enjoyable to drink and can help us relax, but excessive drinking becomes risky quite quickly. Regularly drink more than the government-recommended units per day, or indulge in binge drinking, and you could be risking serious illness or even shortening your life substantially. See pages 102-4.

FOOD PREPARATION

Some ready-made sauces, microwave meals and takeaways can contain high levels of saturated fat, sugar and salt. Cooking from fresh ensures that you know exactly what has gone into your food and are getting the maximum benefit from it. Cut yourself some slack if your creations don't look the same as they do in that celebrity cookbook you bought. Experiment! Cook alongside your partner, or get the kids to help and make cooking and eating a relaxing social experience. Remember: food is not just fuel; it can affect our wellbeing and happiness in all kinds of ways.

EXERCISE

You don't need to train for a marathon or cycle in the Tour de France: the main thing about exercise is that it should be regular. A brisk ten-minute walk is better than no walk at all, and you can increase the time and effort as you feel able. For an extra burst of incentive, join a group or a class full of people who will notice if you're not there. Those who don't exercise are risking dozens of health problems in old age, ranging from osteoporosis and arthritis through to heart disease and stroke. In fact, most of the health conditions we talk about in this book are improved by regular exercise!

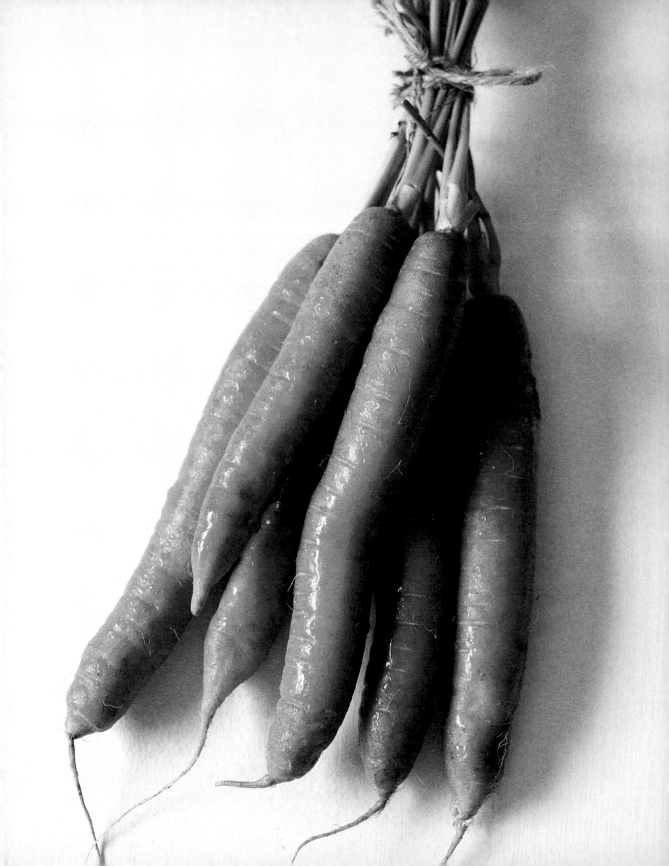

WEIGHT

All the answers to this question score zero because we're making the point that it's not always easy to understand what your weight should be. Read pages 58-60 for more insight into this issue. But be aware that obesity causes and exacerbates most of the life-threatening diseases associated with old age, and will probably mean that you get them earlier than your slimmer friends.

SUN EXPOSURE

The incidence of skin cancer has increased massively in the past twenty years and it's now one of the top ten diagnosed cancers in men and women. Sun beds are particularly risky because of the way the UV rays are delivered to your skin. Don't avoid sun exposure completely because it stimulates our bodies to produce vitamin D. We need 15 minutes per day between May and September to achieve our recommended levels. Children are at risk of rickets if they don't get enough sun, because they are covered at all times by hats and full-strength sunblocks. But be sensible and don't ever overdo it.

ILLNESS PREVENTION

It's important to have regular health checks at your local practice, rather than just turning up in A & E once you are at death's door. Women between twenty-five and sixty-four should be undergoing regular screening for cervical cancer, as recommended by their specialist or GP, and in some circumstances this may start at a younger age. All women over fifty should have regular mammograms, and rectal exams can be useful to identify prostate enlargement in men. You won't know if you have high blood pressure or high cholesterol unless your doctor tests them for you. If you are worried about having your blood pressure checked, tell your doctor beforehand and he or she will make an allowance for what is known as 'White Coat Syndrome' – some people's blood pressure goes up in the surgery and goes down again after they leave! Accept all the health screening appointments you are offered. They were put in place because they save lives.

SALT

Salt has been used for centuries to season food and act as a preservative. Roman soldiers were paid a *salarium* to buy the stuff, which is where the word 'salary' comes from. However, excessive salt is known to raise blood pressure. Your taste buds can get accustomed to having lots of salt in the diet and if you reduce it, food may taste bland. Cut down gradually, give yourself a chance to adjust, and before long you won't notice the difference. Two common sources of salt are processed, packaged foods – which can contain very high levels, even in foods where you wouldn't expect to find any – and salt added at the dinner table. If you cut both from your diet, you'll be doing yourself a huge favour.

Does it feel as if it would be a mammoth undertaking to change your life in all these ways? Well, don't do it all at once. Make three changes at a time. Perhaps you could cut down on your drinking, introduce more fruit and veg to your diet, and take up a new exercise programme; or give up smoking, sunbeds and adding salt to your food. Wait until each change has become a routine part of your life that you do without thinking much before adding further changes. Every little thing you do will help to make you healthier, both now and in the future.

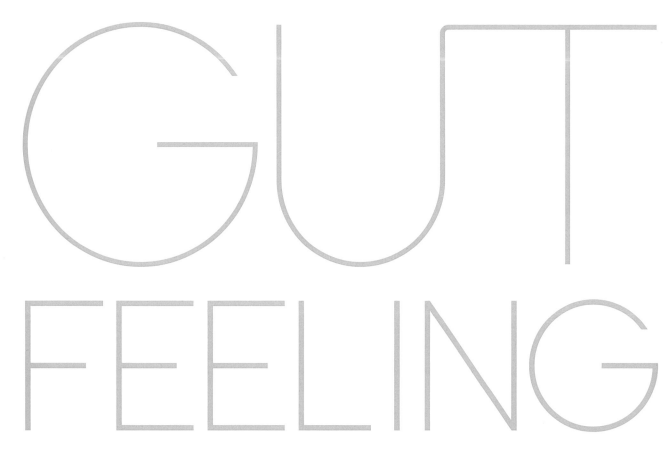

Our digestive system is like a highly specialized factory for extracting energy and nutrients from the food we eat in order to maintain our bodies and keep them functioning on a day-to-day basis. Gut health is absolutely central to our daily, general and long-term wellbeing, and if we don't eat well, we get ill. A huge number of common ailments, including PMS, emotional conditions, memory problems, heart and circulation disorders, chronic colds and, of course, digestive problems, such as constipation, heartburn and IBS, are related to poor gut health, so it makes sense to take care of this very important system.

So, how does it work? The food we eat is chewed and mixed with saliva, which creates a paste that the rest of the digestive system can work with. This travels to the stomach, where it is churned up further and mixed with acid that helps to neutralize any bugs and toxins in the food. Then the food is slowly and gradually allowed into the small intestine for further chemical digestion by the juices of the pancreas and the liver. The food is then broken down into its constituent elements – amino acids found in proteins, vitamins and minerals, various sugars and individual fats – that are absorbed in the small intestine.

After this, food enters the large intestine, where a host of bacteria set to work digesting it further and producing stable waste products that we pass out as bowel movements. Without these bugs, the large intestine does not work effectively and we get symptoms such as diarrhoea or constipation. If we take a course of antibiotics, for example, our 'healthy' bacteria may be wiped out, and our digestion affected; similarly, if we eat a diet that is far too high in sugar, we'll feed the 'bad' bacteria and other pathogens that can cause ill health.

This is a very delicately balanced operation that can be easily disrupted. Our guts can cope with a fair bit of abuse (in the form of unhealthy foods and excessive alcohol, for example) but over time, their function will be compromised and illness will be the result. A healthy, varied diet, with plenty of fresh, whole foods, will provide the nutrients our bodies need for healthy digestion, as well as fibre, which keeps everything going. When our guts are working efficiently, we are much more likely to achieve optimum health on every level.

BAD BREATH

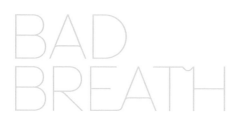

Bad breath *(halitosis)* is not an illness per se but it can be a sign that something is going wrong in the digestive tract. If this is a problem you suffer from, read on for the sake of your close personal friends, as well as for your health.

THE SCIENCE

Bad breath is usually caused by bacteria on the gums, teeth and tongue, and it affects most people at some time in their lives. Those with gum disease are more likely to experience bad breath. Other causes can include digestive problems, such as gastroenteritis or constipation, sinus problems, such as an infection, chronic tonsillitis and tonsil stones, smoking, or eating smelly foods.

Try to work out the cause of your bad breath and treat that. In the meantime, here's some advice you can try to stop people flinching and turning away when they get close enough to smell your breath.

Foods to Eat

- **Green tea** contains polyphenols that have a natural deodorizing effect.
- **Oranges, lemons, limes and grapefruit** – especially first thing in the morning – will help to stimulate the flow of saliva.
- **Fresh mint tea** after a meal is a useful digestif.

- **Chewing parsley** can act as a quick deodorizer.
- **Drink lots of water to avoid a dry mouth.** Fizzy water may help cleanse the teeth and promote saliva flow.
- **Bicarbonate of soda or sea salt in water** will deodorize your mouth and reduce bacteria that can cause odour.

Foods to Avoid

- **Onions, garlic, alcohol, smelly cheese and spicy foods** all cause 'flavoured' breath – but not necessarily bad.
- **Avoid sugary foods with meals (or after),** as they can ferment in the mouth, creating odour; better to eat them before a meal, if at all.
- **Fizzy flavoured drinks and fruit juices** between meals raise the levels of acid in your mouth, causing odour.

Expert Tips

- **Brush and floss your teeth twice a day,** and use a scraper on your tongue (or simply brush it with a soft toothbrush).
- **Change your toothbrush every two months** and visit your dentist every six months.
- **If you smoke,** this is yet another reason to give up.
- **Watch out for very low-calorie or low-carbohydrate diets,** which cause your body to enter 'ketosis' (where your body begins to use your fat stores for energy, creating fatty acids known as 'ketones'). These make your breath smell like pear drops, and some people find it unpleasant.
- **If you get chronic tonsil infections,** see your doctor to rule out tonsil stones.

WARNING

See a dentist if your gums often bleed when you brush your teeth, or if they remain red and sore for more than a week.

See also: Receding gums, Constipation, Sinusitis

BLOATING

Abdominal bloating is a symptom rather than a health condition in its own right. It is characterized by a full, tight feeling in the abdomen, which may be visibly swollen. Causes include being overweight, overeating, swallowing too much air, IBS, acid reflux, food allergies or intolerance, constipation and/or bacterial overgrowth in the bowels.

THE SCIENCE

Bloating is a build-up of gas in the colon, usually caused by an increased production of gas by the bacteria that live there. In some cases, gas builds up (or is over-produced) because of what you've eaten (too much fruit, for example, can give the bacteria a feast, with lots of gas produced as the fruit is fermented), inadequate fibre (so that your bowel movement sits in your colon for longer than it should, fermenting and creating gas), and even stress, which can change the way you digest food. Usually, a change in diet will keep bloating at bay.

Foods to Eat

- **Peppermint tea (or fresh mint in a salad)** may help to encourage healthier digestion.
- **Drink plenty of water,** which will keep your bowel movements softer, plumper and easier to pass.
- **Eat lots of fruits, vegetables, pulses, oats and brown rice;** soluble fibre will keep you regular.
- **Leafy green vegetables, nuts and sunflower seeds** contain magnesium, which helps to keep your gut healthy.
- **Fresh pineapple and papaya** contain enzymes that can encourage digestion (see recipe on page 32).

Foods to Avoid

- **Eggs, bananas, cheese, bread and pasta,** which can lead to constipation and bloating.
- **Some people find resistant starchy carbohydrates** difficult to manage; for example, cooled potatoes, cold rice and cold pasta salad.
- **Refined sugars and alcohol** feed bad bacteria, yeasts and parasites in the gut.
- **Blue and aged cheeses contain mould,** which can encourage bloating.

Expert Tips

- **Keep a food diary** to find out whether any particular foods are triggering your bloating.
- **Chew your foods well.** Lumps of food will take longer to digest in the digestive tract.
- **Don't eat on the run,** which can discourage healthy digestion.
- **Eat little and often** to give your body a chance to digest small quantities of food more efficiently.

WARNING

All bloating that lasts more than a month should be seen by a doctor, particularly if you experience any abdominal pain. It could be a symptom of a much more serious disorder.

See also: Constipation, Coeliac disease, Crohn's disease, IBS, Indigestion

MINTED PAPAYA AND PINEAPPLE FROZEN YOGHURT

Serves 6
Preparation time: 10 minutes
Freezing time: Overnight/24 hours

1. Tip the pineapple, papaya and sugar into the jug of a blender, blend until smooth, add the yoghurt, lime zest and juice and mint, quickly blend to just combine.

2. If you have an ice cream machine, churn to manufacturer's instructions. If not, pour into a freezer-proof container, freeze for 2 hours, return to blender and blitz to break up any ice particles, repeat after 1 hour and then freeze overnight.

Ingredients

300g fresh pineapple, peeled, cored and chopped

200g fresh papaya, peeled, deseeded and chopped

2 tablespoons caster sugar

600g full-fat probiotic yoghurt

grated zest and juice of 2 limes

10g mint leaves, roughly chopped

| Per serving: 131 kcals | 6g protein | 3g fat | 2g saturated fat | 21g carbs | 21g sugar | 2g fibre | 0.2g salt |

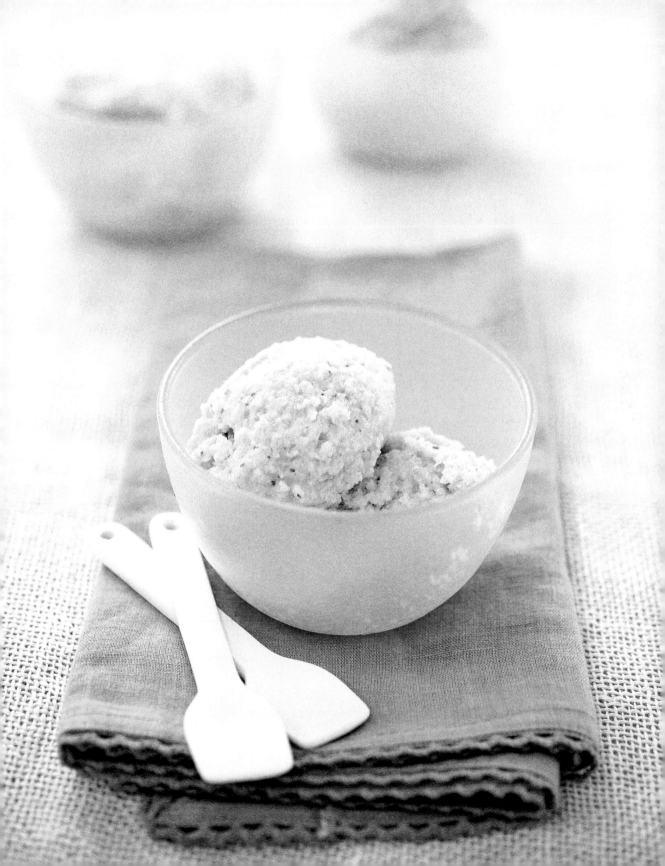

COELIAC DISEASE

Coeliac disease is an auto-immune condition, in which gluten (found in wheat, barley and rye) triggers an allergic reaction. This immune response damages the lining of the small intestine, causing a range of nasty symptoms such as diarrhoea, excessive wind and/or constipation, unexplained nausea and vomiting, stomach cramping and bloating, fatigue and headaches, and iron, vitamin B12 and/or folic acid deficiency. Other symptoms can include weight loss, mouth ulcers, skin rashes, problems with tooth enamel, depression, joint, nerve or bone pain, and hair loss, although these vary between sufferers. Coeliac disease is diagnosed by blood tests, which look for antibodies produced by the body in response to gluten. Sometimes these tests can be inaccurate, and a *biopsy* (taking a small sample of bowel tissue) may be required to confirm a diagnosis.

THE SCIENCE

Gliadin in wheat and similar proteins found in barley and rye appear to be responsible for producing an allergic reaction in sufferers.

Coeliac disease can occur at any time of life, sometimes becoming established after pregnancy, surgery or severe emotional stress. There may also be a genetic link. The only course of treatment is avoiding gluten-containing foods; some grains may be tolerated better than others, and with a dietitian you can experiment to see which you can eat. Try to have as varied a diet as you can manage, to ensure that you get all the nutrients you need; coeliac disease can make it harder for your body to absorb nutrients.

Foods to Eat

- **Choose corn (maize, polenta, etc.), soya, potato, quinoa (see recipe on page 37), cornflour, millet, arrowroot, buckwheat, amaranth and rice flours,** or products to ensure that you get adequate carbohydrates, fibre and B vitamins. There is now a wide range of gluten-free products available, which means that you will be better able to balance your diet.

- **Increase your intake of foods containing B vitamins,** which may be deficient in your diet due to wheat avoidance; these include fortified, gluten-free cereals, leafy green vegetables, meat and eggs.

- **Get plenty of omega 3 oils,** found in oily fish and flaxseed, which can help to ease inflammation.

- **Vitamin C,** found in fresh fruit and vegetables, is important to keep your immune system operating at optimum level.

- **Calcium-rich foods,** such as leafy green vegetables, almonds, dried apricots and soya, should be included if you are avoiding cow's milk products when you begin treatment, or if you have developed a secondary lactose intolerance.
- **Include iron-rich foods,** such as lean meats, eggs, dried fruit and leafy-green vegetables in your diet, to avoid becoming anaemic.
- **Fruit and vegetables** (particularly in their skins) will give you the fibre you need to avoid constipation.
- **Peppermint or other mint teas** can soothe the gut and encourage healthy digestion.
- **Pineapple and papaya** contain enzymes that can help digestion; there is some evidence that people with coeliac disease do not produce sufficient amounts of digestive enzymes.
- **Probiotic drinks and natural yoghurt** can help to encourage healthy digestion and balance of 'good' bacteria in the gut, which can prevent further inflammation and poor absorption of nutrients.

Foods to Avoid

- **Any gluten-containing foods,** such as bread, pasta, cereals, biscuits, crackers, cakes, pastries, pies, pizzas, crispbreads, gravies and sauces, which are not labelled 'gluten-free'.
- **Any grain that contains gluten,** including wheat (wheat flour, wheat starch, wheatgerm, spelt, wheatbran, bulgur wheat, semolina, couscous, etc.), rye and barley (including malted barley). Although oats contain some gluten, they are sometimes tolerated by coeliacs in moderation.
- **Avoid beer and other alcohol** that contains grains; distilled products such as vodka appear to be fine, but drink in moderation to avoid inflaming your gut.

Expert Tips

- **Watch out for 'hidden' gluten,** which can be found in breakfast cereals, some processed meats, dry-roasted nuts, marinades, soy sauce (which may be fermented with wheat), malt, condiments, some spice mixes and much more. It is essential that you read the label on everything you plan to eat.

- **Drink plenty of water** to stay hydrated and prevent constipation.
- **Be aware of the risk of cross-contamination of food.** Ideally, you need to make sure that any implements used to prepare or cook your food are scrupulously cleaned. It's a good idea to keep a separate toaster for gluten-free bread.

WARNING

See your doctor if you experience weight loss or suffer from fatigue. Have regular health checks to ensure that you do not become anaemic or develop osteoporosis.

See also: Anaemia, Constipation, Bloating, Flatulence, Depression, Osteoporosis,

CASE STUDY

Adam was a small baby, but seemed to thrive until he was weaned on to solid foods. He began to lose weight, suffered from chronic diarrhoea, and seemed listless and tired most of the time. His mother kept a food diary, and discovered that his symptoms were always worse after eating pasta and bread. Coeliac disease was diagnosed by a specialist, to whom he had been referred by the family GP. Adam began a strict gluten-free diet, and immediately began to put on weight. He became more energetic, and experienced a growth spurt within a few months of making the changes. Because gluten is found in so many foods, he does occasionally suffer from symptoms, but his mum finds that warm cups of mint tea help to ease stomach pains.

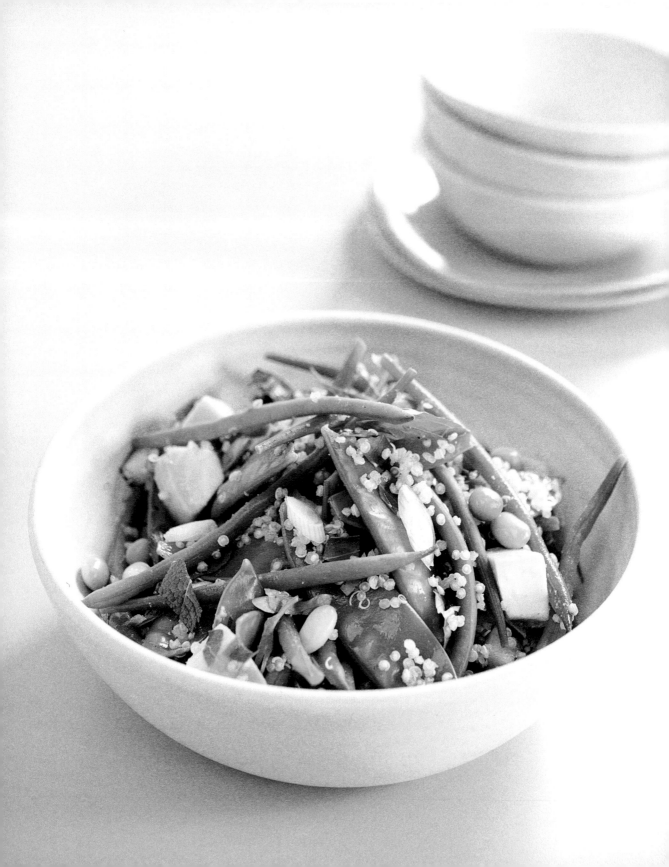

KEENLY
QUINOA
SIDE DISH

Serves 4
Preparation time: 10 minutes
Cooking time: 20 minutes

1. Cook the quinoa according to pack instructions, drain and refresh.

2. Bring a large pan of water to the boil. Add the soya beans, peas, French beans and mangetout or sugarsnap peas and allow to cook for 4 minutes. Drain and refresh in plenty of cold water. Using kitchen towel, pat dry and tip into a large salad bowl along with the quinoa. Add the remaining salad ingredients.

3. Whisk together the dressing ingredients, pour over the salad and use your hands to gently combine well.

Serve with griddled meat, fish or an alternative bean dish.

Ingredients

70g quinoa
100g frozen soya beans
100g frozen peas
100g French beans
100g mangetout or sugarsnap peas
4 spring onions, finely sliced
1 small avocado, peeled and diced
20g mint, chopped
20g flat leaf parsley, chopped
¼ cucumber, diced

For the Dressing

Juice of 1 lemon
1 teaspoon ground cumin
1 tablespoon extra virgin olive oil
Freshly ground black pepper

| Per serving: 184 kcals | 7.5g protein | 10g fat | 2g saturated fat | 16g carbs | 4g sugar | 4g fibre | trace salt |

CONSTIPATION

Constipation is a common condition that can affect people of all ages, and simply means passing stools less frequently than normal, straining more than usual to do so, and finding it difficult to completely empty your bowels. Stools are often hard, dry, large or lumpy. This condition can be short-term, causing no lasting problems; however, chronic (long-term) constipation can be painful and lead to complications. Diagnosis is normally made on the basis of symptoms, but tests may be undertaken to rule out more serious problems.

THE SCIENCE

Constipation is normally caused by having too little fibre and fluid in your diet, although it can also be a side-effect of stress, some medications and health conditions (for example, IBS). A sedentary lifestyle can exacerbate constipation, as can changes of diet (such as when you travel abroad), and it is also common during pregnancy and in babies and children who drink large quantities of milk or begin weaning (as it can take some time for the digestive system to adjust to a new diet). Treatment usually involves increasing your fibre and fluid intake. A laxative (such as psyllium seeds or lactulose syrup) can be used as a temporary measure to keep things moving.

Foods to Eat

- **Fruit, vegetables and whole grains** contain high levels of fibre, and should form the mainstay of your diet. Adults need between 18 and 30 grams of fibre every day, and to get this you need to include fibre-rich foods at every meal.
- **Eat both soluble and insoluble fibre,** which play different roles. Soluble fibre is found in fruits, vegetables, oat bran, barley, seed husks, flaxseed, pulses and soya; insoluble fibre is found in whole grains, nuts, seeds, and pulses (see recipe on page 40).
- **Wheat bran and prunes** both encourage softer bowel movements that are easier to pass.

Foods to Avoid

- **Tea, coffee and colas act as a diuretic,** and can leave you mildly dehydrated, causing constipation.
- **Refined, processed foods** tend to be low in fibre and can exacerbate symptoms.
- **Overeating dairy products** can cause constipation.

Expert Tips

- **Increase your fluid intake;** you should get around two litres of fluid each day (ideally water) to hydrate your system, and keep your bowel movements soft.
- **Get regular exercise** (at least five times a week) to stay regular.
- **Make sure you don't rush bowel movements or hold them in;** respond to your body's natural urges.

WARNING

Report any change in bowel habits to your doctor, particularly if there is blood or mucus in the stool.

See also: IBS, Coeliac disease, Flatulence, Pregnancy

GRANOLA BARS

Makes 15 bars
Preparation time: 15 minutes
Cooking time: 40 minutes

1. Preheat the oven to 180°C/160°C fan/gas 4. Line a 29 x 21cm baking tin with baking parchment.

2. Tip all of the nuts, seeds and oats on to a large baking sheet and toast in the oven for 15 to 20 minutes or until golden. Leave to cool a little. Pulse a few times in a food processor or chop roughly. Pulse all of the dried fruit or again roughly chop and mix with the nut mix.

3. Melt the butter in a saucepan with the honey and sugar over a medium heat. Pour over the fruit and nut mix and stir to combine, spoon the mixture into the prepared baking tin, push down well with the back of a metal spoon and bake for 15 to 20 minutes or until golden. Mark into 15 pieces but leave to cool completely before removing from the tin and cutting into bars.

You could use any combination of nuts, seeds and fruit – mix it up with your favourites.

Ingredients

100g almonds
100g cashew nuts
100g blanched hazelnuts
50g pumpkin seeds
50g sunflower seeds
1 tablespoon milled linseed/flaxseed
1 tablespoon shelled hemp
150g rolled oats
175g dried figs
175g dried dates
150g raisins
175g butter
75g runny honey or agave syrup
125g light brown sugar

| Per serving: 340 kcals | 7g protein | 20g fat | 4.5g saturated fat | 36g carbs | 28g sugar | 4.5g fibre | 0.13g salt |

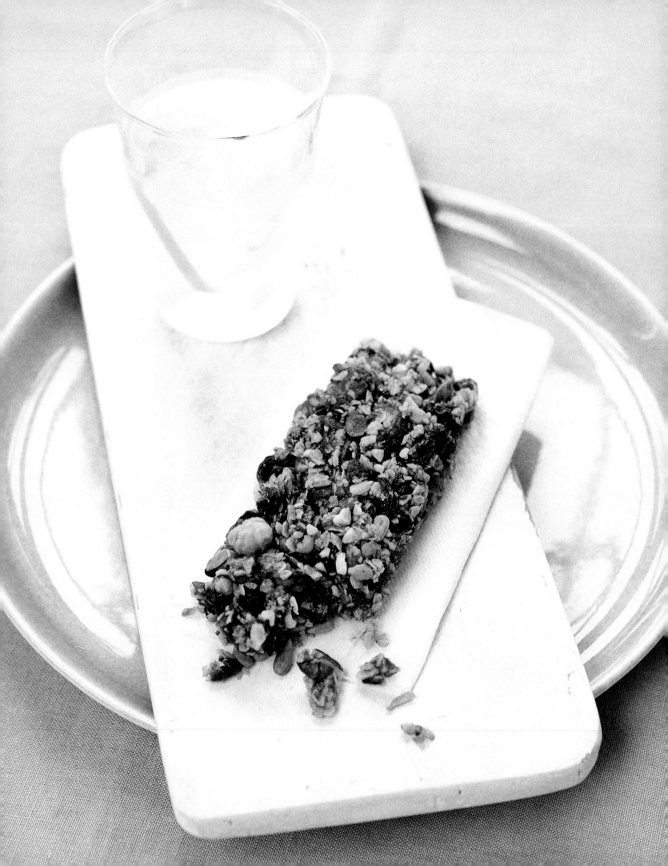

CROHN'S DISEASE

Crohn's disease is a distressing inflammatory bowel disease (IBD), which normally affects the intestines, but can occur anywhere along the digestive tract, from the mouth to the anus. Inflammation makes the intestinal walls thicken, causing a host of symptoms, including abdominal cramping, fever, fatigue, loss of appetite, pain when passing stools, weight loss and persistent, watery diarrhoea. Sufferers may also experience constipation, joint pain, mouth ulcers, swollen gums, skin ulcers and inflamed eyes. There are a number of tests that can confirm diagnosis, including scans, x-rays and internal procedures such as colonoscopy.

THE SCIENCE

The cause of Crohn's is unknown, but there seems to be a genetic link. It may also be triggered by viruses and particular elements in your diet, and stress can worsen symptoms. Treatment involves anti-inflammatory medication, which may need to be taken on a long-term basis to control the condition. Sometimes surgery might be necessary to remove affected parts of the bowel. Crohn's disease can go into 'remission' (which means that it goes away for a period of time), but you will always be susceptible to flare-ups.

Foods to Eat

- **Cooked, easy-to-digest foods** such as vegetable soups and stews can ensure you get the nutrients you need without inflaming the bowel further.

- **Some patients have found that the FODMAP diet** (see page 54) eases symptoms.

- **A low-fat diet** can help to prevent diarrhoea.

- **Make sure you get plenty of calcium-rich foods** (soya products, milk, leafy green vegetables and almonds) to avoid deficiency; this nutrient is often low in people suffering from Crohn's.

- **Iron levels** also tend to be low in sufferers, leading to anaemia; eat plenty of well-cooked lean meats, dried fruit, leafy green vegetables and eggs.

- **Oily fish and flaxseed,** which contain omega 3 oils, can ease inflammation and should be eaten several times per week.

- **Eat foods high in B vitamins, calcium and magnesium,** such as whole grains (if fibre doesn't cause problems for you), dark leafy green vegetables (spinach and kale), and sea vegetables.

- **Antioxidant fruits and vegetables** can encourage healing and reduce inflammation. In particular, orange and yellow fruits and vegetables contain beta-carotene, which is required for the health of your mucous membranes; as the bowel is lined with these membranes, good levels of this nutrient can help.

Foods to Avoid

- **A low-fat low-fibre diet** is easier to digest and doesn't put too much pressure on your inflamed bowels, so avoid eating large quantities of whole grains, pulses or fruit and vegetables and fats.
- **Alcohol** can inflame the digestive system, so avoid or make sure you drink only with meals.
- **Raw vegetables and salads** can exacerbate symptoms.
- **Dairy products** can aggravate symptoms in some people; a lactose-free, low-fat milk may be more easily tolerated, as will live yoghurt.
- **Avoid spicy foods,** refined foods and caffeine, which can make symptoms worse.
- **Eating sugar and processed foods** may make you more likely to develop the disease, and can make it worse in sufferers.

Expert Tips

- **Eat little and often** to keep energy levels up and make digestion easier.
- **Smoking** is a risk factor for Crohn's, so if you smoke, give up as soon as possible.
- **Relax,** get plenty of sleep and take steps to deal with any stress in your life; stress is a major factor in worsening symptoms.
- **Regular, gentle exercise** can reduce stress and help to maintain overall health. Make sure you stay well hydrated during and after exercise.
- **Take a slow-release multivitamin and mineral tablet every day.** Because of decreased appetite, problems absorbing nutrients, chronic diarrhoea and the side effects of medication, you may not get enough nutrients from the food you eat.
- **Spend plenty of time outside in the sunlight,** to encourage your body to increase its stores of vitamin D, which can protect your bones.
- **With the help of a dietitian,** some people respond well to a liquid-only diet to induce and maintain remission.

CASE STUDY

ennifer was diagnosed with Crohn's when she was a student. She suffered from chronic diarrhoea and pain, which she originally believed was due to stress and a poor diet. When Crohn's was diagnosed, she changed her diet completely to cut out all raw fruit and vegetables, sugar, processed foods and fatty meats. She still managed to eat five or six servings of fruit and vegetables each day, but she cooked them well. She also began to eat more oily fish, and sprinkled ground flaxseeds on porridge made with fine oats and soya milk each morning. Jennifer found that eating four or five small meals a day helped her symptoms, as did drinking lots of water. She began to take yoga classes, which reduced her stress levels. She's been in remission for two years now, and has not experienced any flare-ups. Jennifer is convinced that her careful attention to her diet has made all the difference.

WARNING

If you experience fever, blood in your stool or any lower abdominal pain, contact your doctor.

See also: Osteoporosis, Anaemia, Flatulence

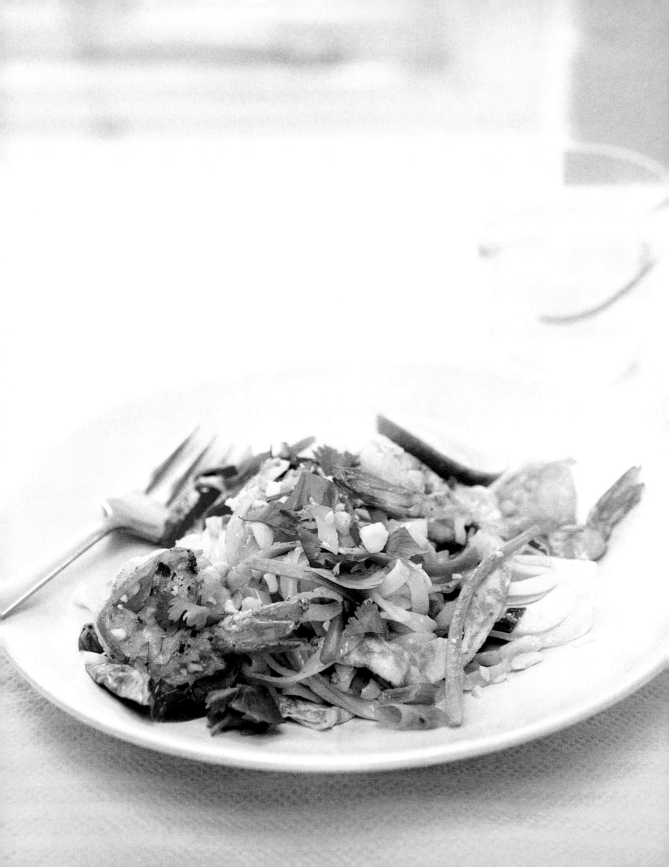

PAD THAI

Serves 4
Preparation time: 20 minutes
Cooking time: 10 minutes

1. Follow the instructions on the packet to soak the noodles, drain and rinse in cold water.

2. Over a high heat, heat half of the oil in a large frying pan or wok, swirl round to coat the sides, pour in the eggs and swirl round, and cook for 1 to 2 minutes until set. Carefully remove the thin omelette from the pan and slice into ribbons similar width to the noodles, set aside.

3. Heat the remaining oil in the same pan over a high heat, tip in the prawns, pepper, pak choy, carrots and spring onions, and stir-fry for 3 to 4 minutes or until the prawns have turned pink throughout.

4. Whisk together the chilli, tomato puree, fish sauce, sugar and lime juice. Add this sauce and the noodles to the pan, stir over a moderate heat for 2 minutes to combine all of the ingredients and reheat the noodles.

5. Gently stir in the omelette and serve immediately, scattered with coriander and peanuts, and with a lime wedge to squeeze over.

Ingredients

200g thick rice noodles

2 tablespoons sunflower oil

2 eggs, lightly whisked

300g raw king prawns

1 red pepper, deseeded and sliced

2 pak choy, quartered

2 carrots, peeled and finely sliced into matchsticks

6 spring onions, green part only, finely sliced

½ teaspoon dried chilli flakes

1 tablespoon tomato puree

2 tablespoons fish sauce

1 teaspoon palm or brown sugar

Juice of 1 lime

20g bunch coriander, roughly chopped

1 tablespoon unsalted peanuts, finely chopped

Lime wedges, to serve

| Per serving: 416 kcals | 23g protein | 12g fat | 2g saturated fat | 54g carbs | 13g sugar | 4g fibre | 2.3g salt |

FLATULENCE

Flatulence or 'passing wind' from the digestive system via the anus is a common and normal process. In fact, most of us pass wind many times a day without even being aware of it. It becomes a problem when it is excessive or very smelly – usually the result of lifestyle or dietary issues.

Some medical conditions can cause flatulence, such as IBS and constipation, but it does not normally require a medical diagnosis, unless there are additional symptoms suggesting a digestive condition.

THE SCIENCE

In most cases, flatulence is simply caused by the foods we eat; for example, a very spicy curry with (or even without) alcohol will cause a change in the bacteria of the colon, and lead to a different type of fermentation – producing more or different-smelling gas. Foods that are more difficult to digest (such as raw fruit and vegetables and whole grains) tend to be only partly digested in the small intestine before hitting the large intestine. The bacteria here literally attack the food to ferment it, and produce lots of foul-smelling gas. It could be that irregular bowel movements are at the root of problem flatulence. Treatment simply involves being more aware of what you eat, and staying well hydrated.

WARNING

Any changes in bowel habits that last more than a month should be reported to your doctor.

See also: IBS, Crohn's disease, Bloating, Indigestion, Coeliac disease

Foods to Eat

- **Cooked fruit and vegetables** may produce less wind than raw.
- **Rice, bananas, citrus fruits, grapes, hard cheese, eggs, nuts and yoghurt** tend to create less gas.
- **A probiotic drink or live yoghurt** can address the balance of healthy bacteria in the gut, and ease flatulence in some people.

Foods to Avoid

- **Eating excessive quantities of very high-fibre foods** may be a problem, so cut down the number of servings of whole grains you are eating each day if you are eating more than three.
- **High-fat food** can generate a large amount of fatty acid, which are released as a pungent gas.
- **Some foods simply produce more gas** because of their structure; these include beans, cabbage, onions, sprouts, cauliflower, broccoli, apples, peaches, pears, corn, ice cream and soft cheese.
- **Fizzy drinks** can contain lots of sugar and additives, which can cause gas throughout your system.

Expert Tips

- **Keep a food diary** for a few weeks and note down any patterns.
- **Chew food thoroughly,** and take your time over meals.
- **Smaller, regular meals** put less pressure on your digestive system, and can ease flatulence.

HAEMORRHOIDS

If you've got haemorrhoids (piles) you'll know all about it, as they can be itchy, painful and awkward to live with (you may also see a little bright red blood when you use toilet tissue). They are swellings that develop in the lining of the anus from engorged veins, rather like varicose veins. There are differing levels of severity, but most haemorrhoids are small and will settle down by themselves. Larger ones will need treatment by your GP or a surgeon.

THE SCIENCE

Pressure and straining seem to be the main factors in developing haemorrhoids, though the exact reason why they form is still unclear. For the moment, avoiding pressure is the best advice, and that means avoiding constipation. Don't try to go to the toilet when you aren't ready; don't try and hold it in, either. Pregnant women are prone to haemorrhoids due to pressure in the abdomen reducing the peripheral blood flow, but pregnancy piles should settle down after you've given birth. Getting older, being overweight and family history are other predisposing factors for developing piles.

Treatments range from making lifestyle changes (especially to your diet) and using topical creams (which can help symptoms such as itching) right through to surgery, but most cases of haemorrhoids will respond well to changes in what you eat and how you behave. Introduce more fibre to your diet gradually if you're not used to it.

Foods to Eat

- **Increase your fibre intake to guard against constipation.** Eat wholegrain foods, such as tasty wholemeal bread. Have lots of fresh fruit and vegetables, and eat the skins wherever possible.
- **Choose porridge for breakfast** – oats are high in soluble fibre (see recipe on page 48).
- **Have a few nuts as a snack,** rather than sweets.
- **Drink a lot – mostly water** but fruit juice as well – because you need to keep hydrated.

Foods to Avoid

- **Alcohol** can cause constipation and diarrhoea, and you want to avoid both, so it's worth cutting it out altogether when you have haemorrhoids.
- **Caffeine makes you dehydrated,** so try cutting it right back.
- **Lots of red meat** can cause constipation.

Expert Tips

- **Some iron supplements can lead to constipation.** Ask your pharmacist or GP about alternatives; the same applies to painkillers involving codeine.
- **Don't strain or spend too long on the toilet** as this can worsen your symptoms.

WARNING

About half of the population experience piles at some time so there's no need to be embarrassed about talking to your GP.

See also: Constipation, Varicose veins, Pregnancy

APPLE AND BERRY OATY BREAKFAST

Serves 4

Preparation time: 5 minutes + overnight cooling time

1. In a bowl, combine the oats, water and apple juice. Cover and leave in the fridge overnight. Over a high heat, toast the seeds in a dry frying pan for 1 to 2 minutes, shaking frequently, until they turn golden and begin to pop. Tip into a bowl and leave to cool overnight.

2. In the morning, stir the honey, lemon zest and grated apples into the oat mixture. Spoon into 4 bowls and top with the defrosted fruit, the toasted mixed seeds and yoghurt.

The fruit can be alternated to increase the variety of nutrients taken.

Ingredients

225g whole rolled porridge oats

300ml water (cold)

100ml fresh apple juice (not from concentrated)

60g mixed seeds

220ml natural yoghurt

3 tablespoons runny honey

grated zest of 1 unwaxed lemon

2 apples, peeled and grated

200g mixed frozen berries, defrosted

Per serving: 382 kcals	12g protein	9.5g fat	1g saturated fat	67g carbs	25g sugar	6.5g fibre	0.2g salt

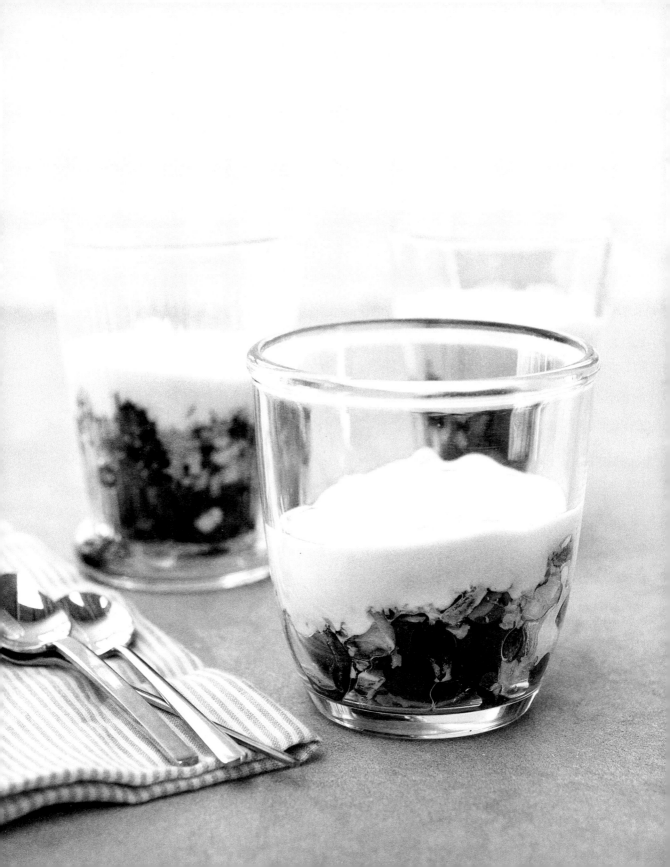

INDIGESTION AND HEARTBURN

Indigestion (dyspepsia) and acid reflux (heartburn) are caused by stomach acid upsetting the upper part of the gastrointestinal system. The acid produced in your stomach is an important component of the digestive process. However, it is really strong and if it is produced to excess (for example, when we are stressed, or in smokers and those with certain illnesses) or is in the wrong place, it can cause significant symptoms. The most common symptom is pain (usually after eating) in the upper abdomen. Reflux – in which stomach acid is regurgitated into the oesophagus, causing burning – can also affect some people. Bloating, wind, burping and nausea may also be present. Most people experience indigestion occasionally, and it is uncomfortable but not usually debilitating.

THE SCIENCE

There are a number of different causes of indigestion and heartburn, including a 'faulty' valve between the stomach and oesophagus in the case of reflux, and inflammation of the stomach (which is responsible for gastric ulcers and some cases of indigestion) that may be caused by diet, stress, alcohol consumption, smoking and the helicobacter pylori bacteria. Gallstones (pebble-like deposits that form in your gallbladder) may also cause a type of indigestion or pain in the upper abdomen that is sometimes mistaken for indigestion. Even something as simple as gulping meals can cause acid problems and being overweight will make you more susceptible.

Foods to Eat

- **Eat protein** (vegetable sources, such as pulses, tofu, nuts and seeds, or animal sources such as eggs, meat, poultry and fish) with every meal. Protein stimulates the gallbladder to excrete bile (which acts to digest food) into the small intestine.

- **Hot peppers contain capsaicin,** which helps to get rid of acid; regular, small amounts of spicy foods may actually improve heartburn (reflux), although they are not recommended for indigestion in general.

- **Healthy fats** – particularly the omega 3 oils, found in oily fish and flaxseed – can soothe inflammation and encourage healthier digestion. Make sure your overall intake of fats is not excessive though. Fat slows the emptying of the stomach, so can make ingestion worse.

- **Raw vegetables** are difficult for the body to digest, and may put your digestive system under too much pressure; you may also fail to digest them adequately to get the nutrients they contain. When symptoms improve, they can be slowly reintroduced.

- **Raw vegetables contain nutrients** such as vitamin C, folate and betacrotene, which can counteract any damage to your gullet.

Foods to Avoid

- **Peppermint, alcohol, fizzy drinks and fats** relax the muscle of the valve between the stomach and oesophagus, allowing stomach acid to flow upwards.

- **Cheese, butter and heavily marbled meats** are high in saturated fats, which can slow down the emptying of the stomach, causing reflux and indigestion. Eat in moderation.

- **Citrus is a trigger** for fifteen per cent of heartburn sufferers.

Expert Tips

- **Keep a food diary** and note down how you were feeling and what you were eating or doing before an attack. By ascertaining the triggers that cause problems, you can take steps to avoid them.

- **Avoid smoking,** which can make the problem worse.

- **Rest, relax and get plenty of gentle exercise,** which can help to reduce stress-related acid problems.

- **Avoid lying down** immediately after eating, and avoid eating before bed.

- **Sleep with your head raised** (putting some books under the head of the bed, for example, or just using another pillow).

- **Sip a little water with meals** to ensure that the contents of your stomach become liquid enough to be passed into the intestines; too much fluid with meals, however, can slow down digestion.

- **Break your daily food intake into five or six small meals,** which are more easily managed by the digestive system. Avoid large, spicy meals.

- **Achieve a healthy weight** – many acid problems are exacerbated by being overweight.

- **Chew foods thoroughly** and slowly to stimulate your digestive enzymes.

- **Avoid overcooking proteins,** which makes them difficult to digest.

WARNING

Report pain, difficulty swallowing or any long-term digestive problems to your doctor.

See also: Stomach ulcers

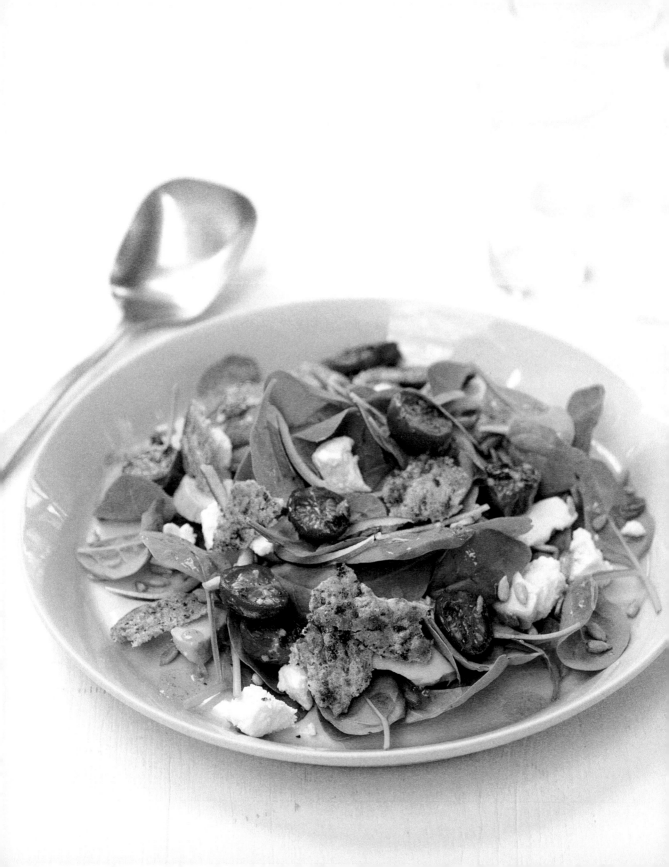

SPINACH SALAD WITH TOMATOES, FETA AND SUMAC CROUTONS

Serves 2
Preparation time: 15 minutes
Cooking time: 35 minutes

Ingredients

1. Preheat oven to 150°C/130°C fan/gas 2.

2. In a large bowl combine the tomatoes, thyme leaves, crushed garlic and olive oil, season with freshly ground black pepper, stir well and spread out onto a small baking try. Place in the oven for 25 minutes or until beginning to wrinkle.

3. Peel the pitta breads apart and place on a second tray sprayed with oil. Liberally spray the pittas and sprinkle them with the sumac.

4. Remove the tomatoes from the oven and put to one side to cool. Turn the oven up to 180°C/gas 4 and cook the pittas for 10 minutes or until golden and toasted. Remove from the oven and break into bite-sized pieces.

5. Tip all of the salad ingredients into a large bowl. Make the dressing by whisking the ingredients together, season to taste with more freshly ground black pepper. Dress the salad, tossing to coat. Sprinkle with the pitta croutons and arrange the tomatoes on top.

200g cherry tomatoes, halved
1 tablespoon fresh thyme, leaves only
1 small clove garlic, crushed
1 teaspoon olive oil
Freshly ground black pepper
2 wholegrain pitta breads
Olive oil spray
1 teaspoon sumac
200g baby leaf spinach
60g feta, crumbled
1 avocado, peeled and sliced
½ red onion, thinly sliced
1 tablespoon sunflower seeds, toasted
1 tablespoon pumpkin seeds, toasted

For the Dressing
2 tablespoons extra virgin olive oil
Juice of 1 lemon
Juice of 1 orange
1 tablespoon sumac

Per serving: 665 kcals | 21g protein | 42g fat | 11g saturated fat | 50g carbs | 13g sugar | 13g fibre | 2.2g salt

IRRITABLE BOWEL SYNDROME

Irritable Bowel Syndrome (IBS) is a chronic (long-term) condition characterized by abdominal pain and discomfort, changes in bowel habits and abdominal bloating. It is very common, affecting between ten and twenty per cent of people in the UK, and can seriously affect their quality of life, although the condition itself does not usually pose a threat to health. Symptoms can include bouts of constipation and/or diarrhoea, excessive wind, an urgent need to pass stools, passing mucus with stools and abdominal cramping. It can also cause lower back pain, fatigue, joint and muscle pain, headaches, bad breath, urinary and bowel incontinence, nausea and burping. Diagnosis is usually made on the basis of symptoms, although a *sigmoidoscopy* or *colonoscopy* can be used to rule out other problems.

THE SCIENCE

There is no clear-cut cause of IBS, which is, simply, a set of symptoms that indicate that your colon is irritated and is not functioning properly. There is some evidence that more frequent or stronger contractions of the muscles lining your bowel may create symptoms, but the reasons for this are unknown. Stress, medication (such as antidepressants and antibiotics) and diet may be at the root of the problem for some people; in other cases, there is no clear-cut cause. In most cases, changing your diet will reduce, alleviate or even eradicate symptoms. You may require mild laxatives, antispasmodic medication, anti-diarrhoea medicine and painkillers during attacks.

The FODMAP diet has proved a resounding success for many sufferers. The term FODMAP is used to describe a collection of carbohydrates that are found in many foods (it stands for Fermentable Oligo-, Di- and Mono-saccharides and Polyols). The theory is that eating foods that are high in FODMAPs results in increased levels of liquid and gas, causing distension and symptoms such as pain, gas and bloating. Generally speaking, foods that are high in fructose (fruit sugar) and lactose (milk sugar) are considered to be high-FODMAP foods; rye and wheat in large quantities are the same.

High-FODMAP foods include apples, apricots, cherries, mangoes, pears, nectarines, peaches, plums, watermelons and tinned, dried and juiced fruits. Custard, ice cream, all types of animal milk, margarine, soft cheese and flavoured yoghurt, as well as baked beans, chickpeas, lentils, kidney beans, corn syrup, artichokes, asparagus, avocados, beets, broccoli, Brussels sprouts, cabbage, cauliflower, garlic, fennel, leeks, mushrooms, okra, onions, peas, shallots and sugarsnap peas are also high-FODMAP.

Low-FODMAP foods include bananas, blueberries, grapefruit, grapes, honeydew melons, kiwi fruit, lemons, limes, oranges, raspberries, strawberries, maple syrup, butter, hard cheese, lactose-free milk and ice cream, rice milk, sorbet, carrots, celery, corn, aubergines, green beans, lettuce, parsnips, tomatoes, spring onions (green only), gluten-free products and spelt.

Basing your diet around low-FODMAP foods can make a big difference to your symptoms; it's perfectly acceptable to eat those that are higher, but in moderation and singly, rather than with other high-FODMAP foods. You'll find out more about the diet at *www.fodmap.com*, but never self-prescribe it. Check with a qualified dietitian, who can assess your individual case and tailor an eating plan accordingly.

Foods to Eat

- **Probiotic drinks and live yoghurt** can relieve IBS symptoms, posssibly by improving the general health of your gut.
- **Oily fish and flaxseed** are high in omega 3 oils that can help to ease any inflammation present.
- **Choose foods that are low in fibre** during bouts of diarrhoea, and then foods that are higher in fibre if you experience constipation.
- **Mainly low-FODMAP** foods (see above).
- **Peppermint** has been shown to improve symptoms.

Foods to Avoid

- **Caffeinated drinks,** such as tea and coffee, alcohol and fizzy drinks, all of which will irritate the gut.
- **Foods high in insoluble fibre,** such as whole grains and cereals containing bran.
- **No more than three portions of fruit a day,** eaten before or between meals rather than after.
- **Sorbitol, an artificial sweetener** (also found in chewing gum), which can cause diarrhoea.
- **Processed foods,** which contain a resistant starch that is difficult for your body to digest.

Expert Tips

- **Drink at least two litres of water each da**y to stay hydrated (particularly important during bouts of diarrhoea) and to keep bowel movements regular.
- **Regular exercis**e has been shown to reduce symptoms, keeping your bowel movements regular and reducing stress.
- **Relaxation techniques** are useful for many people, particularly if stress makes symptoms worse.
- **Keep a diary to work out what foods or events in your life create symptoms;** it's very helpful to be able to pinpoint problem areas that can be avoided in future.
- **Eat regular meals,** with snacks between, to keep digestion steady.

WARNING

Any weight loss, bleeding, mucus or chronic diarrhoea should be reported to your doctor.

See also: Crohn's disease, Flatulence, Constipation

SWEET POTATO FRITTATAS

Makes 12 muffin-sized frittatas

Preparation time: 10 minutes

Cooking time: 25 minutes

1. Preheat oven to 200°C/180C fan/gas 6. Using olive oil, grease a 12-hole American muffin tin and put to one side.

2. Meanwhile, cut 12 x 15cm squares of non-stick baking paper. Spray the 12 muffin holes with some olive oil and line each hole with a square of baking paper.

3. In a pan of boiling water, cook the sweet potato for 5 minutes or until tender. Drain and leave to cool.

4. In a large bowl combine the eggs, milk, tuna, sweetcorn, chives and feta and season well with black pepper.

5. Divide the sweet potato evenly between the muffin holes, then spoon over the egg mixture. Sprinkle each frittata with a pinch of parmesan and bake in the oven for 18 minutes or until golden and set. Remove from the oven and leave to cool in the tin for 5 minutes. Serve with low-fat sour cream and chive dip and baby gem lettuce.

Ingredients

Olive oil spray

250g sweet potato, peeled and chopped into 1cm pieces

6 eggs, beaten

75ml full-fat milk

200g tinned tuna in springwater, drained, flaked

1 x 250g tin sweetcorn, drained

1 tablespoon fresh chives, finely chopped

90g feta, crumbled

Freshly ground black pepper

15g finely grated parmesan

Low-fat sour cream and chive dip

Baby gem lettuce leaves, to serve

| Per serving: 129 kcals | 10g protein | 7.5g fat | 2.5g saturated fat | 8g carbs | 2g sugar | 1g fibre | 0.6g salt |

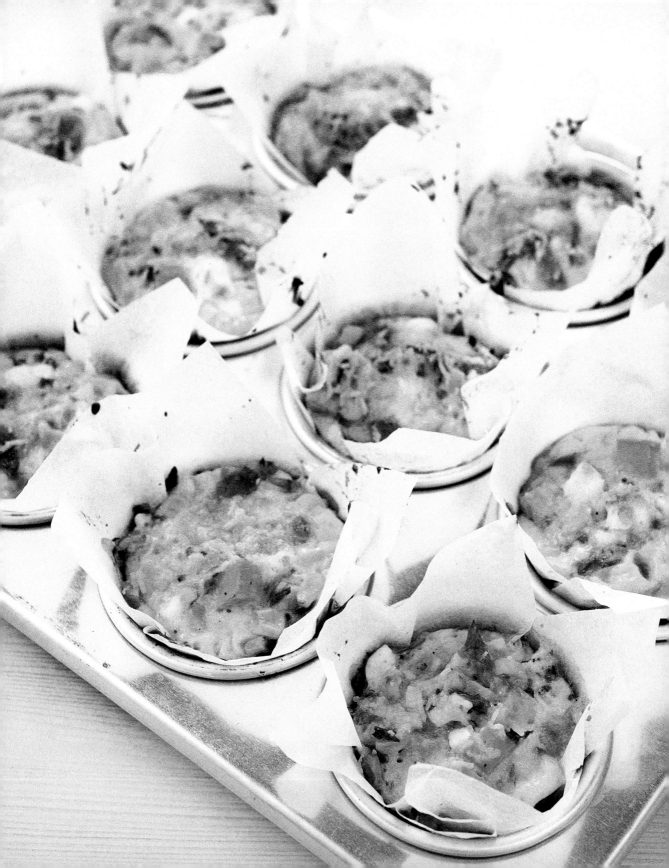

OBESITY AND BEING OVERWEIGHT

Obesity and being overweight can compromise your health on all levels. Just some of the health conditions associated with excess weight include cancer, type 2 diabetes, heart disease, high blood pressure, osteoarthritis, sleep apnoea, kidney problems, gallbladder disease, gout, urinary incontinence – and, of course, low self-esteem. Studies show that most adults are unaware of their exact weight (often under-estimating by more than twenty-five per cent of their body weight), and believe they are 'fit enough', despite statistics showing the opposite. Many of us tend to ignore the scales, and pounds have a habit of creeping on unnoticed. Research shows that menopausal women tend to gain a little over a pound (500g) each year without changing either their diets or exercise habits, and men can pile on the pounds in middle age if they give up regular exercise, such as the Saturday afternoon football match in the park.

THE SCIENCE

Excess weight is, almost always, caused by overeating and under-exercising; in other words, you eat more calories than you burn off. The type of food you eat can also cause you to be overweight; diets high in saturated fat and sugar, as well as those based around processed, refined foods, tend to cause more weight gain than those that include plenty of fruit and vegetables, healthy proteins, good fats and wholegrain carbohydrates. Some of us burn off fat more efficiently (particularly if we exercise regularly and have plenty of muscle). It is also true that our metabolism slows down as we age. Some health conditions can lead to being overweight, including an underactive thyroid gland and polycystic ovary syndrome; however, these are rarer than you may think. Obesity can also be genetic; you are more likely to be obese if your parents are.

Many of us eat not only to fuel our bodies, but for comfort – and even because we have become reliant on certain foods and drinks, such as sugar, chocolate, alcohol and processed foods. We choose foods that quickly raise our levels of serotonin (a chemical in the brain that can ease feelings of depression and anxiety), such as sugary foods and refined carbohydrates; however, these foods also cause spikes in blood sugar and serotonin that can leave us feeling much worse quite soon after eating them. Getting to grips with what and when you are eating – and why – can help you to identify triggers that can be adjusted to create a healthier, more balanced diet.

ARE YOU OVERWEIGHT?

A good way to make a general assessment is to find your BMI (body mass index), which uses a mathematical formula that takes into account height and weight. The chart below will show where you sit on the BMI scale. Generally speaking, a BMI of under 18 is considered to be underweight, 19 to 25 is normal, 26 to 29 is overweight, while anything above 30 is definitely obese. If you've hit a BMI of 40, not only are you considered to be morbidly obese, but your health is at serious risk.

There are drawbacks to this approach, as very muscular fit men and women – and those with very large frames – can weigh more and still be a perfectly healthy weight. Muscle weighs more than fat, so an overweight, slightly built, unfit woman could fall into the normal BMI range, while her fitter colleague may fall into the overweight range.

WEIGHT IN KILOGRAMS / WEIGHT IN STONES

	1.38	1.42	1.46	1.50	1.54	1.58	1.62	1.66	1.70	1.74	1.78	1.82	1.86	1.90	1.94	1.98	
140	74	69	66	62	59	56	53	51	48	46	44	42	40	39	37	36	22s
138	72	68	65	61	58	55	53	50	48	46	44	42	40	38	37	35	21s 10
136	71	67	64	60	57	54	52	49	47	45	43	41	39	38	36	35	21s 5
134	70	66	63	60	57	54	51	49	46	44	42	40	39	37	36	34	21s 1
132	69	65	62	59	56	53	50	48	46	44	42	40	38	37	35	34	20s 10
130	68	64	61	58	55	52	50	47	45	43	41	39	38	36	35	33	20s 6
128	67	63	60	57	54	51	49	46	44	42	40	39	37	35	34	33	20s 2
126	66	62	59	56	53	50	48	46	44	42	40	38	36	35	33	32	19s 12
124	65	61	58	55	52	50	47	45	43	41	39	37	36	34	33	32	19s 7
122	64	61	57	54	51	49	46	44	42	40	39	37	35	34	32	31	19s 3
120	63	60	56	53	51	48	46	44	42	40	38	36	35	33	32	31	18s 13
118	62	59	55	52	50	47	45	43	41	39	37	36	34	33	31	30	18s 8
116	61	58	54	52	49	46	44	42	40	38	37	35	34	32	31	30	18s 4
114	60	57	53	51	48	46	43	41	39	38	36	34	33	32	30	29	17s 13
112	59	56	53	50	47	45	43	41	39	37	35	34	32	31	30	29	17s 9
110	58	55	52	49	46	44	42	40	38	36	35	33	32	30	29	28	17s 5
108	57	54	51	48	46	43	41	39	37	36	34	33	31	30	29	28	17s
106	56	53	50	47	45	42	40	38	37	35	33	32	31	29	28	27	16s 10
104	55	52	49	46	44	42	40	38	36	34	33	31	30	29	28	27	16s 5
102	54	51	48	45	43	41	39	37	35	34	32	31	29	28	27	26	16s 1
100	53	50	47	44	42	40	38	36	35	33	32	30	29	28	27	26	15s 10
98	51	49	46	44	41	39	37	36	34	32	31	30	28	27	26	25	15s 6
96	50	48	45	43	40	38	37	35	33	32	30	29	28	27	26	24	15s 2
94	49	47	44	42	40	38	36	34	33	31	30	28	27	26	25	24	14s 11
92	48	46	43	41	39	37	35	33	32	30	29	28	27	25	24	23	14s 7
90	47	45	42	40	38	36	34	33	31	30	28	27	26	25	24	23	14s 2
88	46	44	41	39	37	35	34	32	30	29	28	27	25	24	23	22	13s 8
86	45	43	40	38	36	34	33	31	30	28	27	26	25	24	23	22	13s 8
84	44	42	39	37	35	34	32	30	29	28	27	25	24	23	22	21	13s 3
82	43	41	38	36	35	33	31	30	28	27	26	25	24	23	22	21	12s 13
80	42	40	37	36	34	32	30	29	28	26	25	24	23	22	21	20	12s 8
78	41	39	36	35	33	31	30	28	27	26	25	24	23	22	21	20	12s 4
76	40	38	35	34	32	30	29	28	26	25	24	23	22	21	20	19	12s
74	39	37	34	33	31	30	28	27	26	24	23	22	21	20	20	19	11s 9
72	38	36	33	32	30	29	27	26	25	24	23	22	21	20	19	18	11s 5
70	37	35	32	31	30	28	27	25	24	23	22	21	20	19	19	18	11s
68	36	34	31	30	29	27	26	25	24	22	21	21	20	19	18	17	10s 10
66	35	33	30	29	28	26	25	24	23	22	21	20	19	18	18	17	10s 6
64	34	32	29	28	27	26	24	23	22	21	20	19	18	18	17	16	10s 1
62	33	31	28	28	26	25	24	22	21	20	20	19	18	17	16	16	9s 11
60	32	30	27	27	25	24	23	22	21	20	19	18	17	17	16	15	9s 6
58	30	29	26	26	24	23	22	21	20	19	18	18	17	16	15	15	9s 2
56	29	28	25	25	24	22	21	20	19	18	18	17	16	16	15	14	8s 11
54	28	27	24	24	23	22	21	20	19	17	17	16	16	15	14	14	8s 7
52	27	26	23	23	22	21	20	19	18	17	16	16	15	14	14	13	8s 3
50	26	25	23	22	21	20	19	18	17	17	16	15	14	14	13	13	7s 12
48	25	24	22	21	20	19	18	17	17	16	15	14	14	13	13	12	7s 8
46	24	23	21	20	19	18	18	17	16	15	15	14	13	13	12	12	7s 3
44	23	22	20	20	19	18	17	16	15	15	14	13	13	12	12	11	6s 13
42	22	21	19	19	18	17	16	15	15	14	13	13	12	12	11	11	6s 9
40	21	20	19	18	17	16	15	15	14	13	13	12	12	11	10	10	6s 4
38	20	19	18	17	16	15	14	14	13	13	12	11	11	11	10	10	6s
36	19	18	17	16	15	14	14	13	12	12	11	11	10	10	9	9	5s 9
	4'6½	4'8	4'9½	4'11	5'½	5'2	5'4	5'5½	5'7	5'8½	5'10	5'11½	6'1	6'3	6'4½	6'6	

An important way of working out whether you are overweight and in danger of experiencing the associated health risks is your waist–hip ratio (WHR). Fat that accumulates around your waist and upper body is considered to be more dangerous than fat that is more evenly distributed, or concentrated on your hips and buttocks. Apple-shaped bodies are associated with higher blood pressure, diabetes and high cholesterol (and a host of other health problems), as well as a poor diet composed of excessive processed food, unhealthy fats and alcohol.

MALE	FEMALE	HEALTH RISK BASED SOLELY ON WHR
0.95 or below	0.80 or below	Low risk
0.96 to 1.0	0.81 to 0.85	Moderate risk
1.0+	0.85+	High risk

You can calculate your WHR by measuring your waist and then dividing it by your hip measurement. So, if your waist is 35 inches (90cm) and your hips are 40 inches (102cm), your WHR is 0.8. Now, check the table above to see whether your WHR puts you at an increased risk of health problems.

Foods to Eat

- **The Eatwell Plate diet** (see page 10) offers a balanced approach to eating, which will help you to achieve a healthy weight. Based on plenty of fresh fruit and vegetables, whole grains, lean proteins and healthy fats, it can help to encourage sensible weight loss without causing cravings or leaving you hungry.

- **Eating low-GL foods** (see page 14) can keep your blood-sugar levels steady, reducing cravings and hunger pangs.

- **A fibre-rich diet** (with lots of fresh fruit and vegetables, whole grains and pulses) can keep you fuller for longer, and encourage maximum absorption of nutrients, making you feel better.

- **Green tea** has been shown to increase your metabolism slightly; sipped regularly throughout the day, it can be a useful aid to weight loss.

- **Blueberries** contain an antioxidant that appears to affect the speed at which we store and burn fat.

- **Protein-rich foods,** such as fish, chicken, nuts, cheese, eggs and pulses, all contain tryptophan, which naturally increases serotonin levels – and keeps them high. It works best when eaten with a small amount of unrefined carbohydrates. Protein is also required for muscle growth, and muscle burns fat.

Foods to Avoid

- **Caffeine** in excess (more than four cups of coffee per day) can make you feel jittery and out of sorts, and encourage overeating.

- **Sugar** may not contain fat, but eaten in excess makes you fat. Any excess sugar in our bodies is laid down as fat (almost immediately), so even if you have an otherwise balanced diet, overeating sugar will cause the pounds to pile on.

- **Saturated fat** in moderation is fine, but it is a calorie-dense food that will cause obesity if you eat too much. Fat is quickly added to your existing fat stores if there is too much in your diet.

- **Refined and processed foods** negatively impact on your blood sugar, leaving you edgy and tired.

- **Alcohol** has almost as many calories as saturated fats, and causes a blood-sugar imbalance that can affect your mood and sleep patterns, and cause cravings.

- **Fizzy drinks** – even diet ones – stimulate the appetite.

Expert Tips

- **There is no 'one-size-fits-all' approach that will work for everyone.** You need to look at your lifestyle (including your exercise habits, the amount of alcohol you drink, your stress levels and the amount of sleep you get), the role food plays in your life (for example, do you use it for comfort?) your food associations (does eating make you feel happy? – keep a food diary) and your existing diet. To lose weight and sustain weight loss, you need to develop a programme that is individual for you – one that you can continue indefinitely.

- **Avoid fad diets,** which may cause initial rapid weight loss, but are, ultimately, unsustainable. Instead, adapt your diet to ensure that it is balanced and healthy, and, most importantly, enjoyable.

- **Make sure you get enough sleep.** People who have less than six hours sleep or more than eight hours per day are less likely to achieve weight loss.

- **High stress levels also affect weight loss.** When combined with poor sleep, stressed people are about half as likely to be successful at weight loss as their less stressed counterparts who get between six and eight hours of sleep. Try relaxation techniques.

- **Don't forget breakfast!** Not only does it kickstart your digestion and metabolism, but you'll be less likely to experience cravings and overeating.

- **Eat three regular low-GL meals per day** to keep blood-sugar levels steady and encourage healthy digestion – don't skip meals.

- **Exercise!** This is the single most important element of weight loss. Not only does it increase your levels of fat-burning muscle, but it raises your 'feel-good' hormones, burns calories and fat, improves the health of your heart and circulatory system and provides an outlet for adrenaline caused by stress.

- **Drink plenty of water.** Dehydration can make you feel hungry, when in fact it is thirst that needs to be sated.

- **Set realistic goals.** You may want to lose several stone in a couple of months, but no healthy diet will allow you to achieve that – and keep the weight off. Better to aim for a weight loss of one to two pounds (500g to 1kg) per week, which is healthy and sustainable.

- **Wear clothing that fits**. Baggy clothing with elasticated waistbands will stop you realizing you have a problem.

CASE STUDY

When Patricia divorced, she began to suffer from anxiety and felt regularly depressed. She found comfort in eating – particularly at night, when the children were in bed – and she soon found herself very overweight. She began keeping a food diary, noting when she was eating and linking it to her moods. She noticed that when she was tired and lonely, she tended to snack on sugary foods and simple carbohydrates, washed down with far too much wine. Knowing her 'trigger' foods and moods made her feel more in control, and she changed her evening routine to include some exercise instead of watching TV. Instead of cutting out snacks altogether, she chose a handful of seeds and nuts, hummus and fresh vegetables, and fresh fruit. As the weight fell off she felt more positive and in control and with her self-esteem soaring, she was able to embark on a regular exercise programme.

WARNING

Any sudden weight gain should be reported to your doctor; if you do fall into the danger zone for BMI or WHR, talk to your doctor about potential health risks.

See also: PCOS, Menopause, Thyroid problems

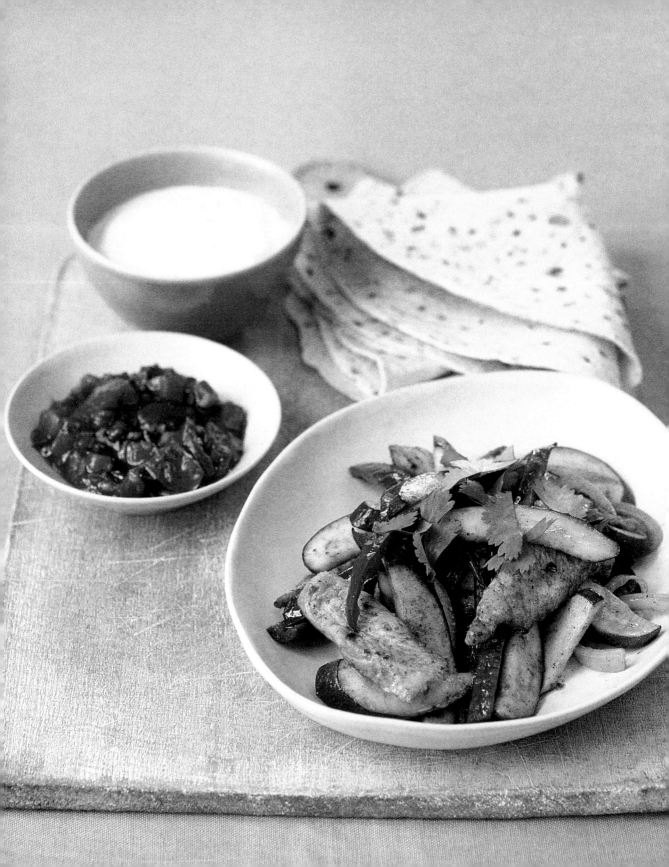

TURKEY AND VEGETABLE FAJITAS

Serves 4
Preparation time: 10 minutes
Cooking time: 10 minutes

1. In a large mixing bowl, combine all of the ingredients and coat well in the oil and spices.

2. In a large, very hot frying pan, fry the turkey and vegetables in batches for 5 minutes each, or until golden and cooked throughout.

3. Warm the tortillas as per packet instructions and serve filled with the turkey and vegetables.

Ingredients

30g packet of good-quality fajita seasoning mix

1 tablespoon olive oil

300g skinless turkey breast, thinly sliced into strips

1 small aubergine, cut into small sticks

1 medium courgette, sliced

4 mushrooms, sliced

1 red or yellow pepper, deseeded and sliced

1 medium onion, thinly sliced

To Serve

8 wholegrain/seeded tortillas

Low-fat salsa

Low-fat crème fraîche

Fresh coriander leaves

Per serving: 406 kcals | 27g protein | 5g fat | 1g saturated fat | 67g carbs | 6.5g sugar | 6g fibre | 1.8g salt

STOMACH ULCERS

Stomach ulcers occur less frequently now that we know that most of them are caused by a bug called *helicobacter pylori* that we can treat with antibiotics. They cause burning, gnawing pain, usually after meals but sometimes before meals. Occasionally they settle down on their own but more often they recur. If you report this to a doctor he will order an endoscopy test at which the ulcers can be seen and diagnosed. Stomach ulcers and duodenal ulcers look just like mouth ulcers, but occur lower down the gut, and they can be accompanied by indigestion, heartburn, vomiting and loss of appetite.

THE SCIENCE

We don't quite know how the *helicobacter pylori* bug gets into the human stomach, but it is thought that we acquire it in childhood from people who have it already. It may be passed in vomit or saliva. In the Far East, where people eat with chopsticks and share communal food bowls, the incidence of this bug goes up to thirty per cent, compared to less than fifteen per cent in the UK. It's treated with a trio of antibiotics to kill the bug, after which the ulcers tend to go away.

Foods to Eat

- **Healthy fats,** such as those found in oily fish, nuts, seeds, flaxseed and olives and their oil, can ease inflammation.

- **Broccoli and Brussels sprouts** contain an antioxidant known as 'sulforaphane', which acts as an antibacterial agent – improving results of treatment addressing the *helicobacter pylori* infection that may be at the root.

- **Green tea** can also inhibit the growth of the *helicobacter pylori* bacteria.

- **Cranberry** contains potent polyphenol antioxidants, which are antibacterial (see recipe page 67).

- **Foods rich in beta-carotene** (found in bright orange and yellow fruits and vegetables) support the health of the mucous membrane lining your digestive system.

Foods to Avoid

- **Curries, salty and vinegary foods** will all irritate ulcers.
- **Alcohol** can damage the lining of your stomach, and also encourage acidity problems.
- **Fried food or chocolate** may increase symptoms.
- **Processed and refined foods** exacerbate acidity problems, as do onions, citrus fruits and tomatoes.
- **Caffeine** can exacerbate symptoms; drink no more than two cups a day.

Expert Tips

- **Eat several small meals** throughout the day, and avoid over-eating at one meal.
- **Make sure you are relaxed before eating,** and that you take steps to deal with any stress in your life; many ulcers are exacerbated by stress and anxiety.
- **Avoid eating within three hours of bedtime.**
- **If you take antibiotics** to address the *helicobacter pylori* bacteria, follow with probiotics to rebalance the healthy bacteria in the gut.
- **Smoking** has been shown to delay healing and cause symptoms to become worse; quit now.
- **Avoid nonsteroidal anti-inflammatory drugs**, including aspirin and ibuprofen, which can cause stomach ulcers, and discourage healing.
- **Milk and cream;** although they can initially neutralize acid, excessive quantities can change stomach emptying and adversley affect your ulcers.

WARNING

See your doctor if symptoms do not improve with changes to your diet, or if you experience any bleeding, nausea and/or vomiting alongside.

See also: Heartburn

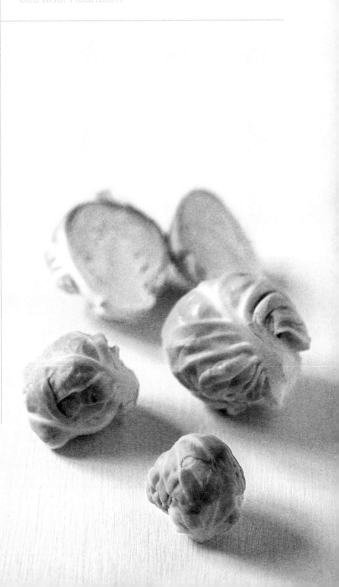

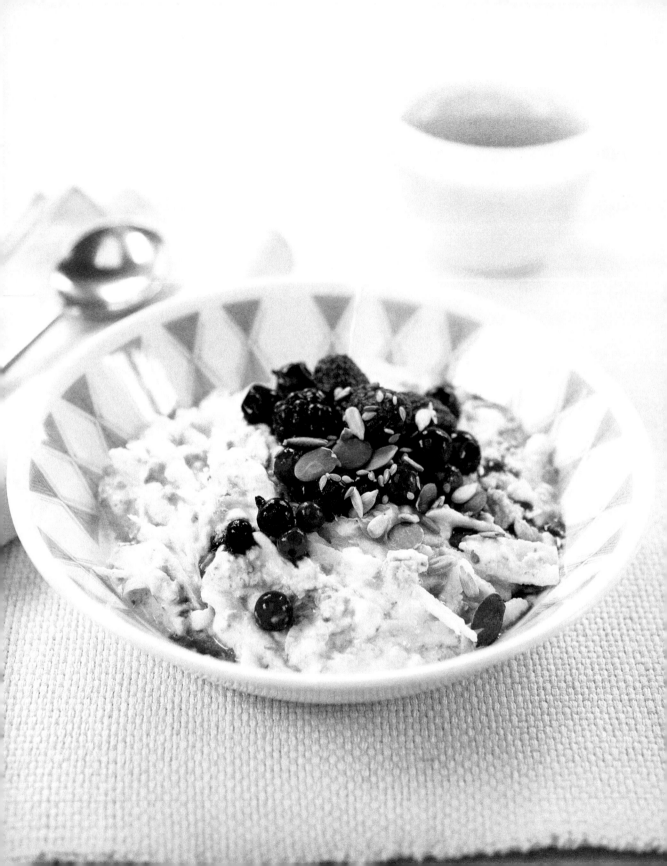

YOGHURT AND BERRY SUNDAE WITH HONEYED OATS AND ALMONDS

Serves 4
Preparation time: 10 minutes
Cooking time: 20 minutes

1. Preheat the oven to 180°C/160°C fan/gas 4.

2. Place the dried cranberries in a small pan along with the apple juice and bring to a gentle simmer until the cranberries are plump, remove from the heat and pour into a small bowl to cool. Stir the cherries and blueberries into the cranberries.

3. Scatter the oats and almonds on to a large baking sheet sprayed with oil and toast in the oven for 10 minutes or until just turning golden. Drizzle with 1 tablespoon of the honey and return to the oven for 6 minutes. Set aside to cool.

4. Stir 1–2 teaspoons of honey into the yoghurt, depending on how much of a sweet tooth you have. Once the oats and almonds are cool enough to handle, tip out on to a large chopping board and roughly chop.

5. In tall sundae glasses or bowls layer the fruit, oaty almond mixture and yoghurt. Serve for breakfast, brunch or as a dessert.

Ingredients

40g dried cranberries

50ml apple juice

150g cherries, halved and stones removed

150g blueberries

For the Topping

Vegetable oil spray

4 tablespoons rolled oats

100g almonds

1 tablespoon runny Manuka honey or other high-antioxidant honey

For the Yoghurt

450g probiotic natural yoghurt

1–2 teaspoons runny Manuka honey or other high-antioxidant honey

Per serving: 391 kcals | 14g protein | 19g fat | 3g saturated fat | 43g carbs | 30g sugar | 4g fibre | 0.82g salt

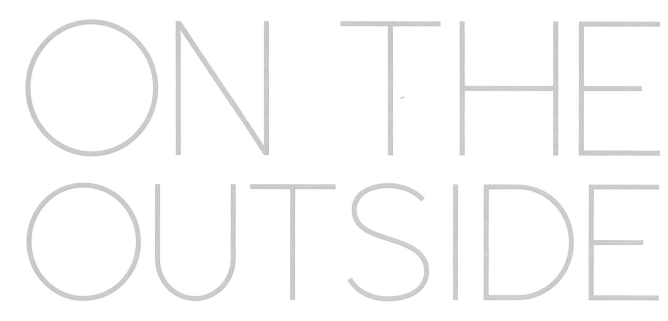

Our bodies don't always give us clear warning signs that there's something wrong. You can have a heart attack at the age of fifty-five without ever having missed a day of work through illness if you have undetected high blood cholesterol levels. By the time you get symptoms of some kinds of cancer, it can be quite late in the day. But our skin, hair and nails can give an external indication that some body systems are not working as efficiently as they might, and it's well worth paying attention to them.

Is your hair thinning, or do you even find clumps of it on your pillow in the morning? It's important to work out why. Do you have ridges or white spots on your nails, a sore mouth or tongue, or changes in your eyesight? Is your skin prone to breakouts or irritable rashes? All of these are signs of something going on within, whether it's a deficiency in an essential vitamin or mineral, a result of normal hormonal changes or, in the case of some skin problems, an allergic reaction.

Some people rely on blood tests to pick up nutritional deficiencies but, while they have their uses, they can give an incorrect impression. A blood test wouldn't pick up a calcium deficiency, for example, because the body maintains a consistent level of calcium in the blood whether or not it's getting enough in the diet, by drawing extra calcium from the bones. You could be well on the way to getting osteoporosis without it showing up in your blood serum.

Eating a well-balanced, varied diet that includes all the nutrients your body requires is the best way to avoid deficiencies, but if you notice external signs that there could be something wrong, don't dismiss them. Pay attention and take steps to deal with them before they get a chance to become more serious health problems.

ACNE

Acne can be very upsetting, whether you suffer from it mildly or are living with a severe case and have blackheads, pustules and cysts all over your shoulders, chest and back. It can leave some sufferers feeling withdrawn and depressed, especially teenagers for whom 'image' and appearance are all-important. But there's no need to suffer in silence, because there's plenty that you and your doctor can do to alleviate the symptoms. And don't ever think you're alone: around eighty per cent of us will experience some form of acne between the ages of eleven and thirty.

THE SCIENCE

Getting acne has nothing to do with poor hygiene; it is primarily related to hormonal changes. Small sebaceous glands just under the surface of the skin produce sebum, an oily substance that keeps the skin smooth. Pores allow the sebum to reach the skin surface, but they can become blocked and bacteria then colonize the area, causing the pustules and inflammation characteristic of acne. Around puberty, levels of androgen hormones surge, causing overproduction of sebum. This is why people often develop acne in their late teens and

early twenties, and is also why it almost invariably improves as they get older.

There is no quick fix for acne and you may need to stick with a treatment for some time to see results. In the first instance, your doctor is likely to recommend a face wash that contains substances like salicyclic acid or benzyl-peroxide, which will remove the old dead skin cells. If this doesn't make enough difference, you may be prescribed a course of antibiotics – either as a cream or in pill form. Some oral contraceptives can help reduce acne in women. If you have a very severe case you may be prescribed retinoid drugs, which work by increasing the production of skin cells and forcing out blockages in the pores. If you do take these, you will need to be carefully monitored as there can be side effects.

Foods to Eat

- **Acne is not caused by poor diet,** but eating a healthy, balanced diet with lots of multicoloured fruits and vegetables and aiming for foods that are low-GL can help to balance your hormone levels.

Foods to Avoid

- **People with acne are often told to avoid eating chocolate, chips or fatty fried foods,** but there's no evidence that they aggravate the condition. You might decide to cut down on them anyway to improve your general health.

- **Reduce the amount of dairy products you eat,** as there is a possibility that could help. Dairy products contain hormones from cows, sheep and goats that may affect our own hormone balance. Don't cut dairy completely because adolescents with growing bones need the calcium they supply, but cut down on it for a few weeks to see if it makes an impact. If there's no change, then reintroduce it.

- **Avoid touching your skin** – and definitely do not squeeze, poke or prod spots! This can spread bacteria and can even cause scarring.

- **Keep your face clean** and wash off your make-up before you go to bed to help unblock pores.

- **Don't fall for internet scams** about miracle products; you'll only waste your money.

- **Eat healthily and get lots of sleep.** Teenagers need more than the six to eight hours that are recommended for adults.

WARNING

Acne is not life-threatening but it can cause severe depression in teenage sufferers, so GPs will always take it seriously.

See also: Eczema, Cold sores

LUCY'S SPAGHETTI BOLOGNESE

Serves 4
Preparation time: 10 minutes
Cooking time: 1 hour 15 minutes

Ingredients

1. Heat the oil in a large saucepan or casserole dish, add the onion and cook over a medium to low heat, covered, for 8 to 10 minutes or until soft and translucent but not browned. Add the garlic to the pan and cook for a further 2 to 3 minutes. Tip in the remaining vegetables and turn the heat up a little, cook for 3 minutes, remove from the pan with a slotted spoon and set aside.

2. Return the pan to the heat and add the beef mince, fry over a high heat, stirring often, for 5 minutes or until the meat is browned. Return the vegetables to the pan and add the chopped tomatoes, tomato puree, chilli and stock, bring to a gentle simmer and simmer part-covered for 45 minutes until the meat is tender.

3. Add the kidney beans and lentils to the pan and simmer for a further 10 to 15 minutes until the kidney beans are softened.

4. Remove the pan from the heat and stir in the olives and basil leaves. Serve with wholegrain spaghetti, cooked as per instructions.

You shouldn't need to add any extra salt to the Bolognese due to the addition of the olives.

2 tablespoons olive or rapeseed oil
1 onion, finely chopped
2 garlic cloves, crushed
1 red pepper, deseeded and diced
1 small courgette, deseeded and sliced
6 button mushrooms, roughly chopped
300g minced lean beef
1 x 400g tin chopped tomatoes
2 tablespoons tomato puree
1 teaspoon chilli powder or flakes
150ml low-sodium beef or vegetable stock
1 x 300g tin kidney beans, drained and rinsed
1 x 400g tin lentils, drained and rinsed
50g chopped, pitted green or black olives
20g bunch basil, leaves picked and roughly torn
Freshly ground black pepper

To Serve
Wholegrain spaghetti

| Per serving: 318 kcals | 25g protein | 15g fat | 4g saturated fat | 23g carbs | 8g sugar | 9.5g fibre | 0.8g salt |

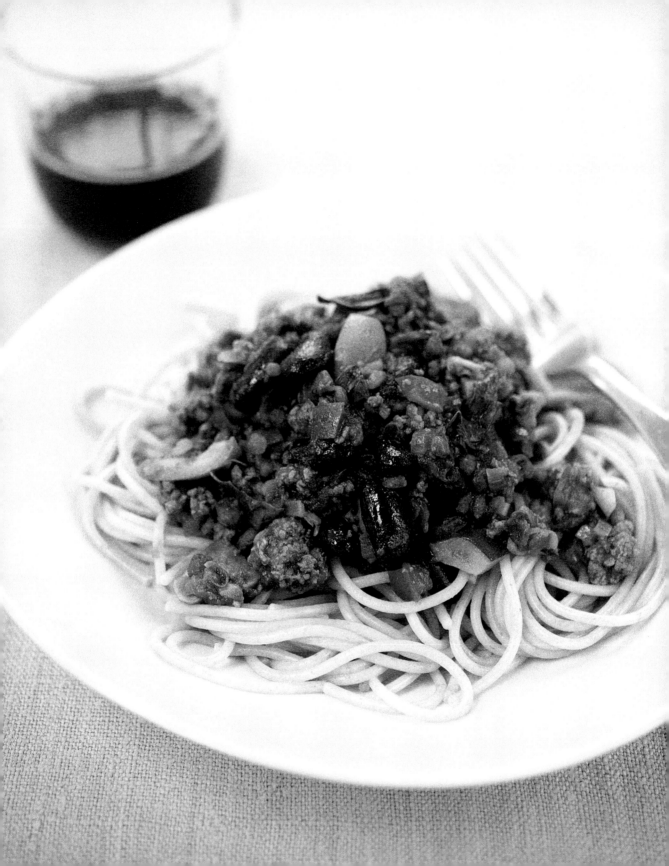

BODY ODOUR

Everyone over the age of puberty has body odour; it's just that some people seem to have more than most, especially around the armpits and feet. And men have more of a problem than women, because they generally sweat more.

THE SCIENCE

There are millions of sweat glands in the human body, and they fall into two types. Apocrine glands are concentrated in the armpits, genitals and breasts and release pheromones – chemicals that have a sweet scent. The sweat they produce is very easy for bacteria to break down, at which point it can start to smell offensive. Bacteria also break down the odourless sweat produced by eccrine sweat glands, which are spread all over the body, but they do it more slowly. The sweat from eccrine glands can take on an unpleasant smell, depending on what you've eaten, because as the body digests certain foods, they release chemicals that are excreted in the sweat. Some foods are worse than others, but it's usually a temporary problem, albeit embarrassing. The smell almost always disappears if you have a shower, though it can return (especially if you put on clothes that have already been worn).

Deodorants just cover up smell with fragrance, but antiperspirants can help to reduce the amount of sweat you produce. Keeping your armpits and feet clean and dry and therefore relatively free of bacteria will help, as will wearing natural fibres which let the skin breathe. Body odour can also be affected by being overweight, as overweight people are likely to sweat more.

If your problem is severe and you can't control it yourself, see your GP. There are treatments that can prevent excessive sweating, including surgery and Botox injections to block the signals from the brain to the sweat glands.

Foods to Eat

- **A healthy, balanced diet,** based on the Eatwell Plate.
- **Drink plenty of water** to replace fluid lost through sweating.

Foods to Avoid

- **Very spicy foods,** curries and those containing cumin and other strong spices.
- **Garlic and onions are common culprits,** producing an acrid body odour.

- **Alcohol and caffeine have been linked to an increase in body odour.** If you think they may be affecting you, try cutting out the booze, coffee and tea for a while and see if this has an impact.

WARNING

If your sweat suddenly starts to smell different, and you haven't eaten anything unusual, check it out with your doctor. Some serious conditions can affect the smell – sweetish sweat can be an indicator of diabetes, for instance.

See also: Bad breath

COLD SORES

Cold sores are irritating, unsightly – and highly contagious. These blister-like spots around the mouth or under the nose are caused by the herpes simplex virus (type 1) and many people catch them as babies when they are kissed by someone with a cold sore. Herpes simplex virus type 2 causes genital herpes. Once again, it is highly infectious and is caught through unprotected sex with someone who has an outbreak.

THE SCIENCE

Once you've been exposed to the herpes simplex virus it remains inactive most of the time. Attacks tend to be triggered when your immune system is weakened, either by another infection or by stress, so if you're under a lot of pressure you may get an attack of cold sores – just what you don't need!

Cold sores usually start with an itchy tingling on the lip, and at that stage you can treat them with over-the-counter cold sore creams containing acyclovir. Most cold sores clear up in about a week.

The most obvious symptom of genital herpes is the presence of painful blisters on the genitals, accompanied by a burning sensation. If you're experiencing anything like this, it's vital you see your GP; genital herpes responds well to regular anti-viral drugs. Don't be embarrassed about seeking treatment. It's part of life, but it's important that you're tested for other STDs or STIs, because if you've caught one infection, you are more likely to have others, some of which can be symptomless.

Note that people with type 1 herpes cold sores on the lips should avoid oral sex during an outbreak.

Foods to Eat

- **Fresh fruits and vegetables** are important to boost your immune system with vital micronutrients. Eat as wide a range of different colours as you can to get all the antioxidants your body needs.

Foods to Avoid

- **There's some anecdotal evidence that avoiding arginine-rich foods,** such as nuts, beans and seafood, can help. Try cutting them out one at a time to see whether they reduce the incidence or severity of your cold sore outbreaks. If there isn't any improvement, you can start eating them again.

Expert Tip

- **Avoid touching your cold sores except when you're applying creams.** Wash your hands frequently with soap and water – and be careful about contact between your cold sores and anyone else's skin. The virus can be transmitted in this way.

WARNING

Frequent severe outbreaks should be checked out by your doctor as there may be other more serious conditions causing the problem.

See also: Eczema, Hair loss, Psoriasis, Stress

DANDRUFF

Dandruff may be unsightly and embarrassing, but it isn't catching and it can be treated effectively. There are lots of things you can try, from anti-dandruff shampoos and simple nutritional tips through to steroid treatments for severe cases.

THE SCIENCE

Skin is constantly being renewed all over the body, but most of the time we don't notice as old cells are pushed to the surface and detach themselves. With dandruff, this renewal happens more quickly: more dead cells are shed, and they are much more obvious as they form clumps.

There are different causes of dandruff. Seborrhoeic dermatitis, which makes the skin become flaky and inflamed, is thought to be caused by a yeast infection. Hormone changes can cause dandruff, and that's why it can be common in teenagers. And a fungus called *Tinea Capitis* is often implicated. If you have this type of dandruff, it will get worse in winter because ultraviolet light stops the fungus growing.

Medicated shampoos can help, as can those containing tea-tree oil, but using lots of hair products such as gels or hairsprays can make it worse. Brush your hair regularly and wash it at least three times a week, but avoid using hair dyes which could irritate the skin. Making sure your diet contains plenty of folate, B vitamins and omega 3 essential oils can help in most cases, but if you have severe dandruff and/or seborrhoeic dermatitis, your GP may prescribe steroid treatments for your scalp.

Foods to Eat

- **Eat lots of whole grains,** green vegetables, nuts, eggs, fish and organ meats to keep up your levels of B vitamins and folate.
- **Oily fish, avocados, nuts,** seeds and olive oil are good sources of omega 3.

Expert Tips

- **In a small study involving twenty people who suffered from dandruff,** Manuka honey (which has anti-bacterial and anti-viral properties) was diluted in a little warm water, applied to the scalp and rubbed in gently for two or three minutes. It was left on for three hours and then rinsed off. All the participants found their dandruff had disappeared. They repeated the treatment once a week for six months and none of them showed any signs of a relapse. You never know – it might be worth a try!
- **Get plenty of fresh air** and sunlight on your scalp. Don't cover up with a hat.
- **Try to avoid stress,** which could make dandruff worse.

WARNING

If you suddenly notice a lot of flaking skin and you haven't had dandruff before, or you have but it cleared up years ago, talk to your GP. Its appearance could be a sign of something more serious.

See also: Eczema, Hair loss, Psoriasis, Stress

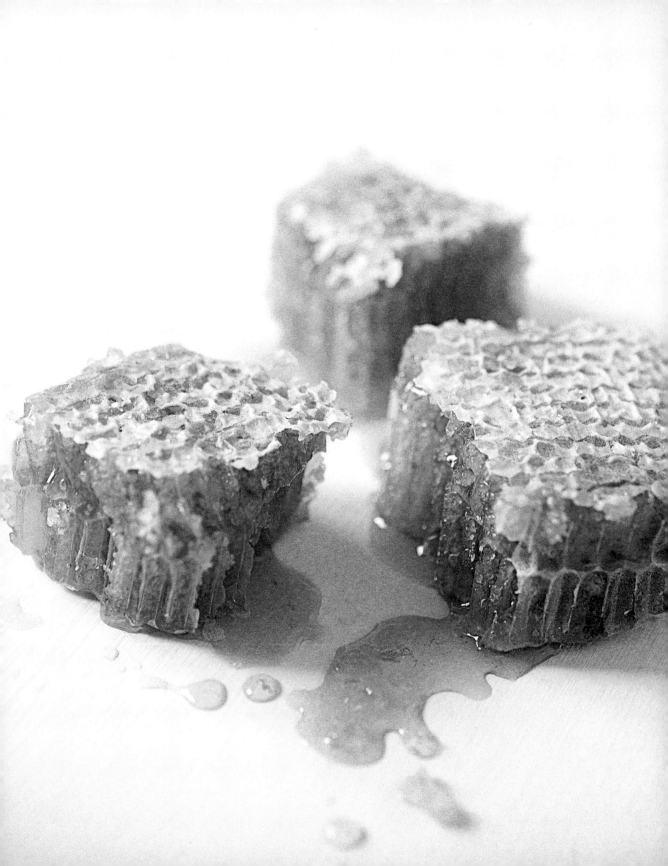

ECZEMA

The red, dry, inflamed and itchy rash of atopic eczema can make life miserable. You want to scratch but know that you can't because it will only make things worse. The good news is that eczema often improves as you get older – up to one in five children get eczema, but more than half grow out of it by their teens. And most people are able to control their eczema with a combination of treatment from the doctor and good management at home.

Contact allergies are responsible for a form of eczema known as contact dermatitis. This is an angry red rash that can develop when your skin is in contact with something you're allergic to, such as the nickel button on a pair of jeans. If a rash appears in one location only, it may be because of something your skin's been touching. Protect yourself from direct contact with the substance (for example, in the case of a jeans button, you could coat the back with nail varnish), and the rash should settle down.

THE SCIENCE

No one knows what causes atopic eczema; it can run in families, but it also seems to be linked to allergies, fluctuating hormone levels and the immune system. Stress plays a part, because it affects the immune system; as a result, eczema tends to get worse when you're under pressure. Eczema overlaps with a lot of other immune-related diseases, and is often associated with asthma. One thing that is certain is that you can't catch eczema from someone else.

Sometimes it is possible to identify triggers that make your eczema flare up. These could be environmental, such as detergents, particular fabrics (wool can be a culprit), skin lotions (especially those that contain lanolin) and perfumes. Stress and hot temperatures can trigger eczema, and some sufferers seem to have trigger foods. Wheat, dairy, eggs, citrus fruits and peanuts have all been implicated and it is worth trying an exclusion diet, cutting them out one by one for four weeks each to see if your symptoms improve. Even if they do improve, you should still reintroduce the food after four weeks to see if they get worse again until you are sure you have the right culprit. (Children should only do this kind of exclusion diet under the supervision of a dietitian.)

Scratching makes eczema worse, so treating the symptoms mainly means helping to relieve the itching. There are various types of cream that can be applied, including simple emollient creams to keep the skin moist. These need to be used all the time, not just when your eczema flares up. Inflammation and infections are treated with steroid and antibiotic creams. Sometimes, eczema sufferers are nervous about using the steroid creams but you should be fine using them short-term, so talk to your GP or pharmacist. Steroid drugs can also be prescribed and are safe when used under medical supervision.

Foods to Eat

- **Choose olive oil instead of vegetable cooking oil** to avoid an inflammatory compound known as arachidonic acid that may exacerbate eczema.

Foods to Avoid

- **Arachidonic acid** is also found in fatty red meats, organ meats, egg yolks and sugar, so cut down on all of these.
- **If you think wheat,** dairy, eggs, citrus fruits or peanuts, may be exacerbating your symptoms, try keeping a food diary and excluding them one at a time to see if there are any improvements. Feeling that you're actually doing something positive can be good for your mental wellbeing.

Expert Tips

- **Itching can be made worse** by contact with detergents and soaps, so use substitutes and avoid anything with colourings, perfumes or lanolin (which can actually trigger eczema outbreaks).
- **If you scratch in your sleep,** try wearing cotton gloves. Rough clothing can be irritating and sweating can also make eczema worse, so try to avoid both.
- **Aim for a healthy body weight;** some studies have shown obesity may be a contributing factor.

WARNING

Scratching can damage the skin and lead to infection setting in. See your doctor if the rash starts to ooze fluid or if you get a raised temperature and feel unwell.

See also: Acne, Psoriasis, Stress

CASE STUDY

aren, a twenty-four-year-old bank clerk, had suffered from really itchy patches of skin behind her knees and in the folds of her elbows ever since she could remember. In her twenties these spread to her chest and face, which made her very self-conscious socially. She tried various herbal remedies without much success and had resigned herself to using cortisone creams and moisturisers, and avoiding soaps. These measures lessened her eczema but never totally got rid of it. She started keeping a diary to see if she could find what triggered flare-ups and noticed that it got worse after she ate oranges and also when she was stressed. She started avoiding oranges and eating kiwi fruit instead to keep up her vitamin C levels, and this seemed to help. She also took steps to deal with the stress levels in her life and within a few weeks of the new regime, the eczema disappeared from her face and chest. She still has it on her knees and elbows but it's much milder and she worries about it a lot less.

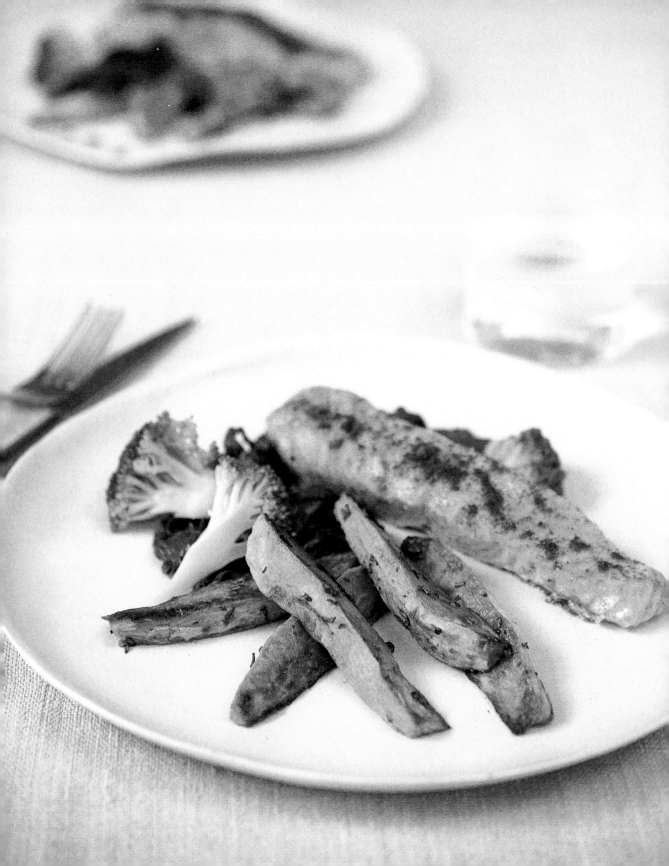

CUMIN SALMON WITH SWEET POTATO WEDGES

Serves 4
Preparation time: 10 minutes
Cooking time: 45 minutes

1. Preheat the oven to 180°C/160°C fan/gas 4.

2. Scrub the sweet potatoes and slice into wedges. Liberally spray with the olive or rapeseed oil spray. Tip the wedges into a large plastic food bag along with the rosemary and garlic. Seal the bag and rub to evenly coat the wedges in the oil, rosemary and garlic. Tip the wedges out on to a pre-heated baking sheet and roast on the bottom to middle shelf for 45 minutes or until browned and tender.

3. While the wedges are cooking, line a baking sheet with foil and lightly spray with olive or rapeseed oil spray.

4. Rinse the fish and pat dry with paper towel. Place the fish with the skinned side down in a single layer on the baking sheet. Combine the spices in a small bowl and sprinkle over the fish.

5. Once the wedges have nearly finished roasting, add the fish to the oven on the middle to top shelf and roast for 10 to 12 minutes, or until the fish flakes easily when tested with a fork.

6. Serve the salmon with the wedges, broccoli and spinach for extra folate punch!

Ingredients

For the Wedges

1kg sweet potatoes
Olive or rapeseed oil spray
4 sprigs rosemary, leaves removed and finely chopped
2 cloves garlic, crushed

For the Salmon

4 x 125g skinless salmon fillets
½ teaspoon ground cumin
½ teaspoon medium chilli powder
¼ teaspoon paprika
Freshly ground black pepper

To Serve

Blanched broccoli
Wilted spinach

Per serving: 313 kcals | 27g protein | 15g fat | 2.5g saturated fat | 17g carbs | 0.6g sugar | 2g fibre | 0.15g salt

HAIR LOSS

It's a fact: nearly all men will lose some or all of their hair over time. There's a hereditary element, so if your father lost his hair by the age of forty, there's a good chance that you will too – but if your grandfather had a full head of hair at eighty, then you could be in luck.

The main reason why most people lose their hair is male-pattern baldness – and women can develop it as well, despite the name. It usually follows the same pattern: a receding hairline, then hair thinning out on the crown of the head and at the temples. Many men find that their hair loss either slows down or stops completely as they get to retirement age.

Male-pattern baldness only affects the hair on your scalp. Alopecia, another cause of hair loss, can mean losing the hair everywhere on your body, though not everyone with alopecia is this seriously affected. If the hair on your head starts coming out in patches, see your GP: it could be alopecia.

An underactive thyroid can also make your hair fall out, as can losing weight suddenly – another reason why it's best to try to reduce your weight gradually. Also, chemotherapy often leads to temporary hair loss.

Whatever the cause, losing your hair can really lower your self-esteem, whether you're male or female, and support groups can be useful for anyone who has problems with it. It can be particularly traumatic for women, but there is help available, so do ask.

THE SCIENCE

Male-pattern baldness got its name because it's related to the 'male' hormone testosterone, but testosterone levels are usually normal in someone who's losing their hair in this way. What happens is that the hair follicles convert testosterone into dihydrotestosterone, which can cause them to shrink, and as they shrink each new hair is thinner than the one before until they become so short and fine that they don't appear above the surface of the skin. There's some work being done which suggests that reducing the level of testosterone will help, and there are drugs which can block the conversion of testosterone, so talk to your GP if you're worried about it. Drug treatments are only effective while you are using them, though. Women who experience male-pattern baldness should always get themselves checked out, as it could be a sign of having raised testosterone levels due to polycystic ovary syndrome.

Alopecia can strike at any age, but most sufferers have their first run-in with it in their teens or early twenties (alopecia can come and go). Some aspects of alopecia are still unexplained, for example, we don't know why only some parts of the scalp are affected. About twenty per cent of alopecia sufferers have a relative who has also had it at some point, so there may be a hereditary element. It's believed to be an auto-immune disease, one in which the hair follicles are attacked by the body's immune system, because it somehow sees them as 'foreign'. This leads to inflammation, the hairs become weak and fall out, and the distinctive bald patches develop. If the immune reaction dies down, the follicles are capable of growing hair again, and in most cases the hair grows back after a year or so.

If you're anaemic, you may be deficient in iron, folate and vitamin B12, and that will affect your hair. If you think this might be the case – perhaps you're feeling very tired and run-down without having a specific reason for being so – ask your GP to refer you for a blood test.

Foods to Eat

- **In some cases, low levels of zinc** have been associated with hair loss. If you eat plenty of seafood (see recipe on page 85), organ meats, eggs, milk and wholegrain products, you shouldn't be deficient in zinc.
- **For folate, eat plenty of dark green leafy** vegetables and legumes.
- **B12 is found in dairy products,** fish, oysters and clams, and liver and kidney.
- **Dark chocolate** is a good source of iron, as are meat, eggs, whole grains and green vegetables.

Foods to Avoid

- **Avoid unhealthy processed food,** as you need to boost your mineral and vitamin levels and these are often low in factory-prepared food. Fill up on the good stuff instead.

Expert Tip

- **Beware of expensive wonder 'cures'** – there are lots out there. Go to your GP first! There are medications he or she can prescribe if male-pattern baldness is causing you great distress.

WARNING

There are lots of possible causes of sudden hair loss. It could be a symptom of lupus or a thyroid condition, as well as anaemia and polycystic ovaries. See your GP if it happens to you.

See also: Anaemia, Polycystic Ovary Syndrome, Stress

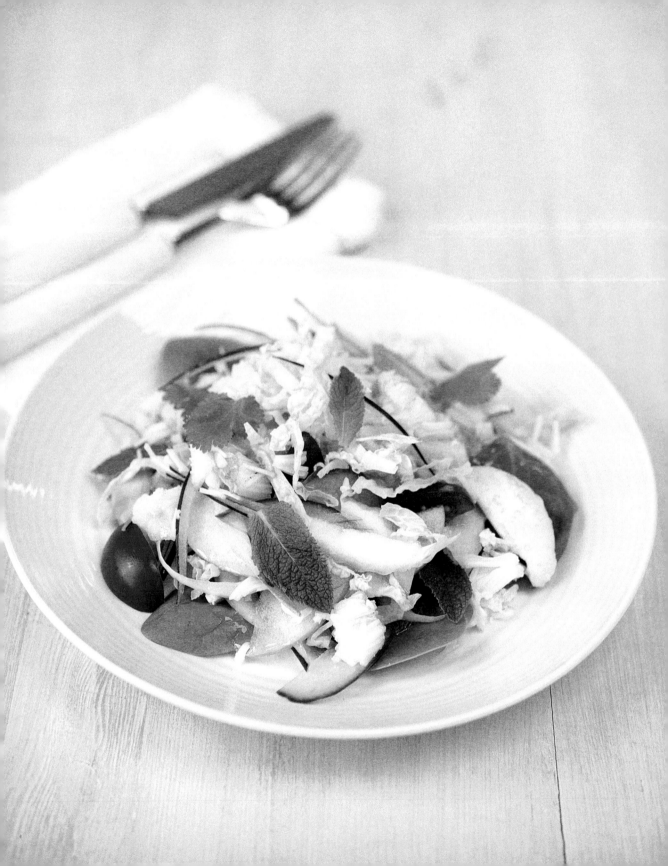

CRAB, AVOCADO AND APPLE SALAD

Serves 4
Preparation time: 10 minutes

1. This salad is so simple to prepare, literally toss together all of the ingredients in a large bowl or platter.

2. Whisk the dressing ingredients together, season with freshly ground black pepper and dress the salad. Simple!

Ingredients

75g baby spinach
75g Chinese leaf, shredded
1 head chicory, shredded
½ red onion, thinly sliced, or 3 spring onions, thinly sliced
½ cucumber, thinly sliced
100g cherry tomatoes, quartered
1 large or 2 small apples, cored and thinly sliced
1 avocado, peeled and sliced
450g fresh cooked crab meat, picked over
20g bunch coriander leaves
10g mint leaves

For the Dressing

Finely grated zest and juice of 2 limes
2 tablespoons extra virgin olive oil
Freshly ground black pepper
¼ teaspoon salt
¼ teaspoon unrefined caster sugar

Per serving: 306 kcals | 24g protein | 19g fat | 3.5g saturated fat | 9g carbs | 7.5g sugar | 5g fibre | 1.2g salt

NAIL PROBLEMS

Nails are made of a hard protein called keratin. Normally, they grow at a rate of up to 5mm a month and the nail beds appear pink while the tips are white, but certain conditions and deficiencies can affect the appearance of nails. It's worth paying attention to weak, brittle nails, white spots or ridges, as they could indicate the lack of some nutrients in your diet.

THE SCIENCE

Problems with nails can be linked to over a hundred conditions, including psoriasis, hypothyroidism and fungal infections, but by far and away the most common thing that damages them is trauma. That could be work-related, gardening or housework – washing up is a prime candidate because it makes nails soft and promotes splitting.

Nutritional causes for nail problems include calcium deficiency, but if you're eating three small portions of dairy food a day – milk, yoghurt, cheese – then that's unlikely. Protein malnourishment can be another cause, so vegetarians and vegans should check that they are eating a wide-enough range of plant proteins. Anaemia, in which you are deficient in iron, vitamin B12 or folate, can cause weak nails, as can not having enough zinc or vitamin A. And having too much selenium can be a problem as well.

Ridges in the nails can be linked to a deficiency in B vitamins in particular, but they can also be caused by stress or being rundown. White spots on the nails could be related to vitamin and mineral deficiencies, but are more likely to be caused by damage to the nail bed affecting its blood supply.

Foods to Eat

- **Remember to eat some dairy three times a day;** this includes the milk you put in drinks or on your cereal. If you opt for dairy substitutes, such as soya milk, make sure they're enriched with calcium.
- **If you're getting enough protein in your diet –** fish, eggs, meat or beans and pulses, nuts and seeds – you're likely to be getting enough zinc and iron, and you'll have plenty of vitamin A if you eat liver.
- **For those B vitamins (B12, folates),** choose leafy green vegetables and whole grains. They'll help with vitamin A, too.

Foods to Avoid

- **Large amounts of carbonated, caffinated drinks** – such as cola – as these can cause increased calcium loss from the body.

Expert Tip

- **Be wary of the supplements designed for healthy nails that you can buy in some pharmacies.** Excess calcium can block the absorption of other essential minerals.

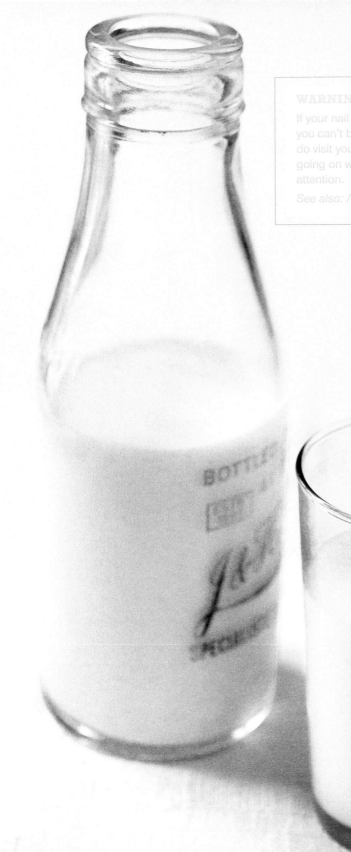

PSORIASIS

Psoriasis is a condition of the skin in which the cells are overproduced, leading to red scaly patches with a silvery appearance. These can be itchy and sore and in severe cases, the skin may crack and bleed. Patches of psoriasis can occur anywhere but typically appear on the outside of the elbows and front of the knee. Some types affect the scalp and the nails, and there is also a form that affects the joints and can cause arthritis.

THE SCIENCE

Psoriasis is an autoimmune gentic condition in which there are high levels of insulin-like molecules that cause the skin cells to grow at a rapid rate, reaching the surface in two to four days rather than the usual twenty-eight days. It has been linked to the metabolic syndrome of insulin resistance. Around forty per cent of sufferers have a family history – and there appear to be triggers for outbreaks, varying from individual to individual. Some people find they occur when they feel a bit rundown; sunburn, cuts and scrapes can bring on an outbreak; alcohol, smoking, obesity and stress are also implicated; and there may be trigger foods as well, which you will have to identify using an exclusion diet.

Treatments include topical creams containing vitamin D and sometimes A, or steroid creams such as hydrocortisone. Keeping the area well moisturized is important to avoid dryness and cracking. A range of medications can be prescribed for severe cases, which will slow down the turnover of skin cells. Regular short bursts of exposure to sunlight can help reduce the inflammation.

Foods to Eat

- **It's important to make sure you get more omega 3s** than omega 6s in your diet, so that means using olive or rapeseed oils instead of vegetable oil and spreads.
- **Some herbs appear to be helpful** because they block inflammatory agents: turmeric, red pepper, cloves, ginger, cumin, fennel, basil, rosemary and garlic are all useful (see recipe on page 90).
- **A vegan diet supplemented with fish oils and vitamin D** may be recommended in severe cases.
- **Lots of fresh fruit and vegetables** increase antioxidants in the body.

Foods to Avoid

- **Arachidonic acid (ARA) is the key** pro-inflammatory component in psoriasis, and it is found in saturated fats, animal fats and sugars. Reducing the quantities of these in the diet may help to reduce the severity of the outbreaks.
- **There's evidence that a gluten-free diet can help.** A blood test can show if you are gluten-sensitive and, if you are, follow the advice for coeliac sufferers (see page 34-5).
- **Alcohol exacerbates psoriasis** and is best avoided altogether if you get it badly.

Expert Tips

- **Use an emollient liquid** rather than soap to wash with, and keep moisturizing to decrease dryness, scaling and itching.
- **Aim for a healthy body weight;** a high BMI can worsen symptoms of psoriasis.

WARNING

Psoriasis is not a life-threatening condition but if it is affecting the quality of your life and making you depressed, then do seek help. It's important to keep your blood pressure in check and consult your doctor about any symptoms that worry you.

See also: Eczema, Stress

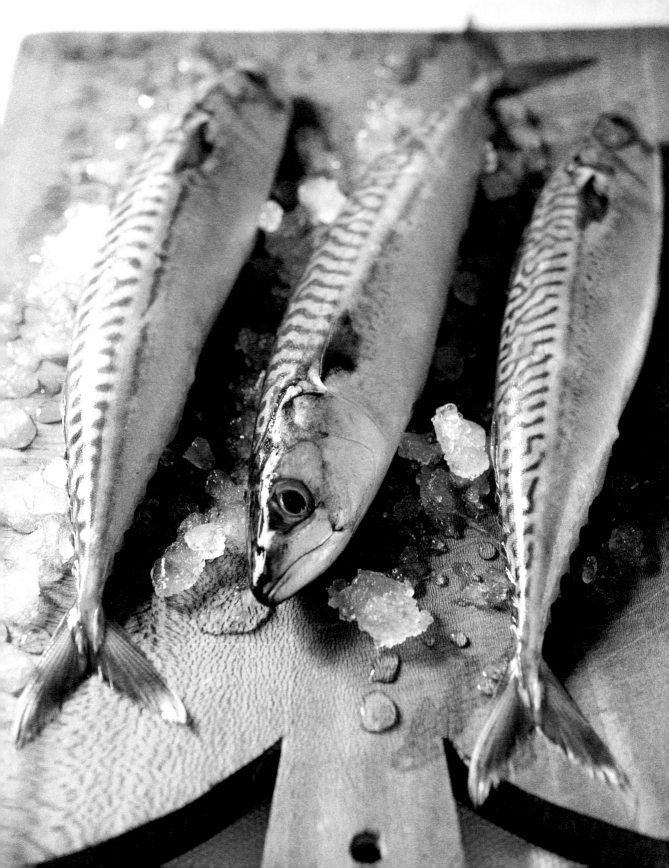

CHICKEN CURRY

Serves 4
Preparation time: 15 minutes
Cooking time: 1 hour 15 minutes

Ingredients

1. Place the onion, garlic and ginger in a food processor and process into a paste. Heat the oil in a large frying pan over a medium heat. Add the onion paste along with a good pinch of salt and fry, stirring continuously, for 10 minutes or until translucent and just beginning to turn golden.

2. Stir in the cumin, turmeric, pepper, cardamom, cinnamon, cloves, bay leaves and nutmeg. Continue to fry whilst stirring for 1 to 2 minutes. Add the chicken thighs and stir them around in the spice mixture until they are well coated and beginning to turn opaque.

3. Pour in the tomatoes along with 100ml water and cover. Reduce the heat to low and simmer gently for 40 minutes. Remove the lid and continue to simmer for a further 20 minutes or until the chicken is cooked through. Remove from the heat, stir through the flaxseeds and season to taste. Serve with rice.

1 large onion, chopped
4 cloves garlic, peeled and chopped
1 slice fresh root ginger
2 tablespoons olive oil/rapeseed oil
Fine sea salt
2 teaspoons ground cumin
1 teaspoon ground turmeric
1 teaspoon ground black pepper
½ teaspoon ground cardamom – this is hard to find so you can use cardamom seeds
2.5cm piece cinnamon stick, broken into pieces
¼ teaspoon ground cloves
2 bay leaves
¼ teaspoon ground nutmeg
8 skinless chicken thighs (grass-fed if possible – higher omega 3 content)
1 x 400g tin chopped tomatoes
1–2 teaspoons flaxseeds (golden linseeds)

To Serve
Cooked rice, optional

| Per serving: 225 kcals | 33g protein | 8g fat | 1.5g saturated fat | 6g carbs | 5g sugar | 2g fibre | 0.4g salt |

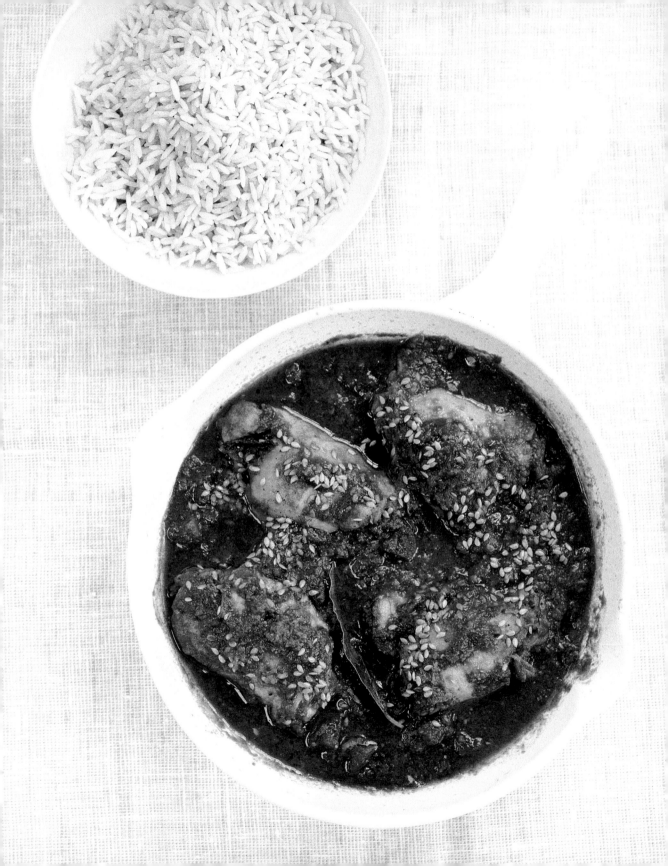

RECEDING OR BLEEDING GUMS

If you smile and more of your teeth are on show than you are used to, or if your teeth seem to be longer or further apart than normal, then you may have receding gums. They're common, but they're not normal – and if left untreated there can be serious consequences, such as teeth falling out. Sometimes receding gums develop so slowly that you might not notice, but they will be picked up if you visit a dentist regularly.

It's easier to spot bleeding gums because there'll be blood on your toothbrush, or when you spit after brushing your teeth. Bleeding gums are a sign of gum disease, usually gingivitis. If it's left untreated it can develop into periodontal disease, and that can also have serious implications and end up with tooth loss. Both receding and bleeding gums can also cause bad breath.

THE SCIENCE

The gums cover and protect the jaw and the sensitive lower parts of the teeth. When your gums recede, this part is exposed and vulnerable, and teeth may feel more sensitive to heat and cold. Aggressive brushing is the commest cause of receding gums. However, poor brushing and poor oral hygiene may lead to excessive plaque build-up and bacterial inflammation of the gums (gingivitis). Inflamed gums are more likely to bleed. Soft plaque can be removed by brushing your teeth correctly twice a day and flossing between them nightly; a dentist or hygienist will remove hardened plaque (known as calculus) at your regular check-ups.

Gingivitis, the main cause of bleeding gums, is also caused by plaque, and can usually be treated by paying attention to dental hygiene. Gums can be prone to bleeding during pregnancy because of all the hormone changes but they should settle down afterwards. Smoking can make the condition worse, as can stress and a poor diet. A diet high in carbohydrates and sugary foods encourages the formation of plaque, and if you eat this way you could have vitamin and mineral deficiencies, which can be another cause of gum problems.

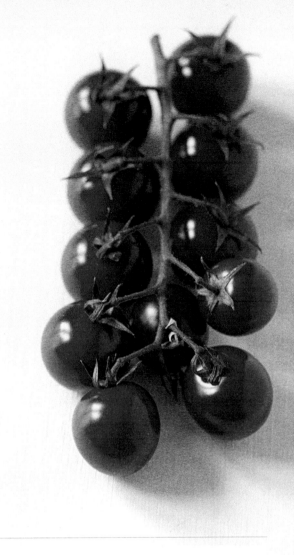

Foods to Eat

- **Lack of vitamin C can be a cause of gum disease,** so eat plenty of fruit and vegetables, especially those high in vitamin C: red peppers, tomatoes, broccoli, kale, spinach, carrots, oranges, mango, canteloupe melon, berries, kiwi fruit.

- **Vitamin K deficiency is less common** but can also be a cause, perhaps if you have a condition that is affecting absorption of nutrients in the gut. K is found in green vegetables, cheese, pork and eggs.

Foods to Avoid

- **Sugar and sugary snacks,** sweets, chocolates, cakes and buns.

- **Fruit as a snack** – have it at mealtimes instead, and brush your teeth 30 to 60 minutes afterwards.

- **Fizzy drinks and fruit juices** can be acidic, and that's not good either. Cut out sugar in hot drinks, too.

Expert Tips

- **Snacking between meals is bad** for your gums as well as your waistline; regular small amounts of sugar can encourage plaque to build excessively.

- **If you are not sure if you are brushing your teeth correctly,** ask your dentist or hygienist for their advice.

WARNING

Any gum bleeding or swelling should be checked out by a dentist or doctor as there are some serious but uncommon causes.

Gum disease increases the risk of developing heart disease. Bacteria enter the bloodstream by way of sore gums, and increase the blood's tendency to clot.

See also: Cardiovascular disease, Bad breath

ROSACEA

It's quite normal to blush or have flushed cheeks sometimes; everyone does! However, if you're having a lot of unexplained flushing and finding that your face stays red for a while, you may be developing rosacea. You might also see small red spots and blood vessels appear. It's common, especially in people with fair skin, and affects women more than it does men. While there's no cure for rosacea, it can be managed and controlled quite effectively.

THE SCIENCE

Nobody knows what causes rosacea, but there's been a lot of work done on what can trigger it and make it worse. Sunlight is a common trigger. Obviously, it's not practical to stay out of daylight for ever, but take sensible precautions. Try using a high-factor sunscreen, but monitor the effects because skin-care products can sometimes cause flare-ups. Stress is another trigger, and so is vigorous exercise. Some sufferers report that relaxation techniques can help, so yoga or meditation are worth trying. Then there are the things you eat and drink. Alcohol comes top of the food and drink trigger list, followed by hot and spicy food. It may be because they increase the blood supply to the skin, leading to flushing, but in some cases there could be an allergic reaction going on. There are medications to treat the symptoms, so visit your GP as well as trying to identify what your own triggers are.

Foods to Eat

- **Eat a healthy, balanced diet,** but monitor it by keeping a food diary and finding alternatives to trigger foods if you need to (for example, if hard cheese makes you flush, try cottage cheese instead).
- **Use herbs to replace hot spices** when you're cooking – substitute coriander and turmeric for chilli and cayenne pepper, for example.

Foods to Avoid

- **Alcohol,** especially red wine, beer and spirits, is the primary trigger.
- **Hot drinks:** tea, coffee, mulled wine, hot chocolate can bring on flushing.
- **Very hot food,** in both temperature and taste, will exacerbate rosacea.

Expert Tips

- **It can be difficult to pin down** triggers for rosacea; some are obvious (alcohol, for instance), but others are less clear. Download a trigger diary from the US National Rosacea Society website: (www.rosacea.org/patients/materials/diary/diarypage.php).
- **If you are a woman aged between forty and sixty,** your flushing could be linked to the menopause. In this case you will feel hot all over when you flush.

WARNING

Over-the-counter medicines for rosacea can sometimes make it worse. In severe cases, the skin can thicken, often on or around the nose. This may need surgery, so it's worth working out your triggers before you reach this stage.

See also: Acne, Eczema, Menopause

VARICOSE VEINS

If you've got lumpy, bumpy varicose veins on your legs or feet, you're far from being alone. They're very common. That doesn't make them any less unsightly, but do be reassured that they're not actually a serious health problem for most people, even though they can be really frustrating – and itchy . . .

THE SCIENCE

When the small valves in our veins stop working as they should, blood can back up and collect in the vein, making it swell. Unfortunately, there's a family tendency to varicose veins, but sensible levels of exercise and controlling your weight can help to mitigate the effects. A sedentary lifestyle doesn't help, and standing for long periods makes them worse (that's one reason why they generally appear on the legs and feet; standing puts additional pressure on the veins there). Pregnancy can also make them worse, and constipation is sometimes another factor.

It's worth talking to your GP if your varicose veins are particularly bad. Treatments can range from compression stockings to surgery, depending on how bad your varicose veins are or whether there are any complications associated with them. If you are simply worried about their appearance, you will usually have to pay for surgery privately. There are procedures that can help, but do some research as they are not all equally effective over time.

Foods to Eat

High-fibre foods help to relieve constipation, and reducing constipation also reduces pressure on the veins, so snack on dried fruit rather than chocolate bars, replace white bread with wholemeal and eat plenty of fresh fruits and vegetables.

Foods to Avoid

Refined foods – white flour, lots of sugar, white rice can all cause constipation, and they don't have the nutrient content of their wholegrain equivalents.

Processed food and ready meals, which are often very low in fibre.

Expert Tips

Keep your weight in the healthy range, because being overweight is a risk factor for varicose veins.

If you have a desk job, make sure you get up and walk around at least once an hour, and if your work means you have to stand up most of the day, it may be worth wearing support tights or socks.

WARNING

Certain herbal remedies – such as horse chestnut and Butcher's Broom – have been associated with an improvement in varicose veins, but be wary. There isn't hard clinical evidence about their efficacy.

See also: Constipation, Haemorrhoids, Pregnancy

WRINKLES/ AGEING SKIN

The way your skin ages is influenced by a combination of genetics and lifestyle. Prolonged sun exposure (especially on fair skin) and smoking are the two worst things you can do for your skin, and wrinkles won't be the worst of the damage they cause either. Good nutrition, drinking plenty of water and using moisturizers all have a role in keeping skin young-looking as long as possible. Some people develop wrinkles earlier than others as a result of habitual expressions – frown lines between your eyebrows, or laughter lines beside your mouth and eyes. But healthy eating over the decades will pay dividends in terms of the appearance of your skin when you reach your sixties and seventies.

THE SCIENCE

The major cause of skin ageing is exposure to the sun; the older you are, the more ultraviolet light your skin will have been exposed to over the years. UV rays damage the collagen and elastin, which keep skin smooth and supple. That's why our hands, neck and face tend to age faster than the skin elsewhere – because they are more frequently exposed to the sun.

Over time, skin becomes more fragile, thinner and less stretchy, all of which make older people more prone to wrinkles. Wearing a sunscreen every time you go out can help to lessen the damage and keep your skin looking younger for longer.

Smokers' skin ages faster than that of non-smokers because the toxins in the smoke actually stop the skin from producing as much collagen. Smokers characteristically get little lines along their upper lips from pursing their lips to suck on a cigarette, and crows' feet at the corners of their eyes from screwing up their eyes to stop smoke getting in. The best thing you can do to put things right is stop smoking. Ensuring that your diet contains a good range of antioxidants and essential fatty acids will help repair some of the damage and prevent more from happening. The Mediterranean diet – with lots of brightly-coloured fruit and veg, not much meat but some eggs and dairy, plenty of whole grains, olive oil – is linked to better skin ageing (and to better all-round health). Dehydration is another element in wrinkling. You need to keep up your liquid intake – water is the best choice – and avoid excessive amounts of anything that might cause dehydration, such as alcohol and caffeine. Moisturizing your skin also helps, and you don't need to spend a fortune on expensive creams. There has been plenty of research showing that a bog-standard skin cream can be just as effective as something more exclusive, as long as it's used regularly.

So, if you want your skin to look its best, protect yourself in the sun with a high-factor sunscreen and avoid unnecessary exposure (such as sunbeds), stop smoking, drink plenty of water and eat well. Stress also affects skin, so take steps to deal with stress levels.

Use omega 3-rich olive and flaxseed oil for cooking or as a salad dressing, rather than vegetable oils containing omega 6.

Avocados, dark green leafy veg, berries, orange-coloured veggies or fruits, pineapple, salmon and tomatoes are all recommended for skin health. Their antioxidant nutrients protect against UV-related oxidation, helping to prevent skin damage (see recipe on page 98).

Keep well hydrated; aim for around 2 litres of water a day.

Saturated fats clog up the system, causing constipation and hardening of the arteries, and the effects of this will be seen in your skin.

Processed food fills you up with non-nutritious mush, meaning you don't have enough room left for essential nutrients.

Keep alcohol and caffeine to a minimum, because they are dehydrating.

Keep your skin moisturized and use a sunscreen if you're in strong sunlight.

WARNING

Any skin blemish that grows rapidly, bleeds, itches or in any way worries you needs to be checked out by your GP.

See also: Eczema, Smoking, Stress

SUMMER ANTIOXIDANT SALAD

Serves 4
Preparation time: 10 minutes
Cooking time: 5 minutes

1. Cut away any skin from the two types of melon and cut into 2.5cm cubes, arrange on a large serving platter, scatter over the pomegranate seeds, feta, olives and onion.

2. Toast the almonds in a dry frying pan over a medium to high heat for 3 to 4 minutes or until golden on both sides, then tip on to kitchen paper to cool.

3. Squeeze the lime over the salad, scatter with the almonds and finish with the herbs.

This salad is great for a lunch or served as a side salad for a BBQ.

Ingredients

½ small watermelon, deseeded
½ cantaloupe melon, deseeded
110g pomegranate seeds
100g feta, crumbled
75g pitted green olives, halved
½ red onion, thinly sliced
50g blanched almonds
Juice of 1 lime
20g bunch mint, leaves only, roughly chopped
20g bunch flat leaf parsley, leaves only, roughly chopped

| Per serving: 270 kcals | 10g protein | 18g fat | 6g saturated fat | 17g carbs | 16g sugar | 3.5g fibre | 1.7g salt |

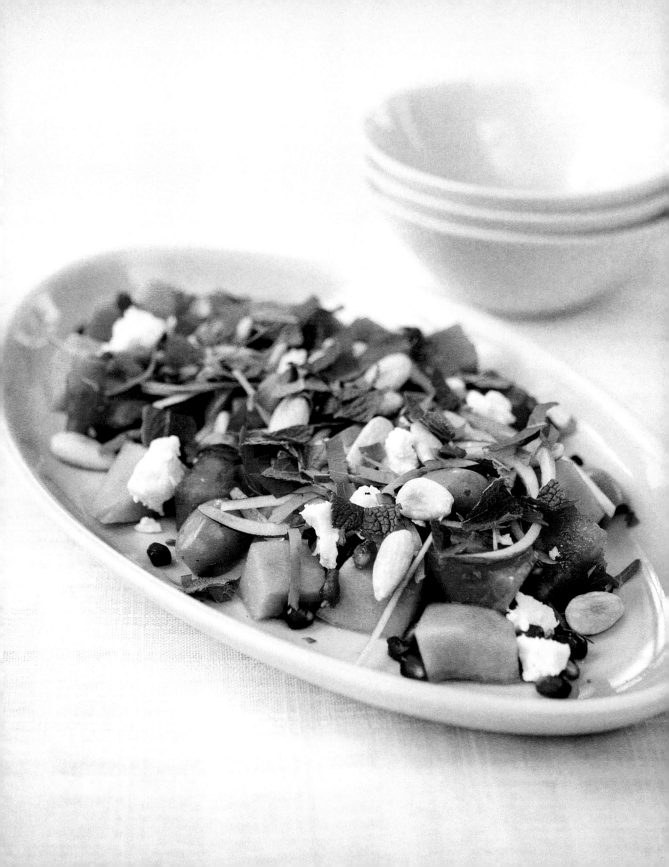

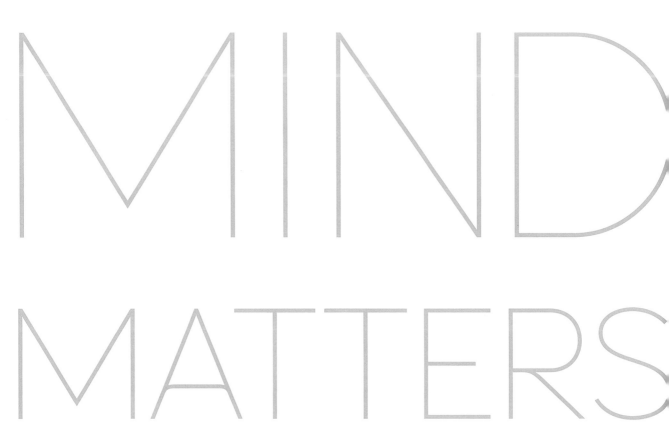

ALCOHOL DEPENDENCY AND PROBLEM DRINKING

Around twenty-four per cent of adults in the UK regularly drink more than the recommended daily units of alcohol. If you are drinking too much, you may think you're getting away with it because there might not be any physical symptoms of liver problems until very late in the day. By the time you wake up with jaundice, your liver disease is pretty late stage and you could be looking at a liver transplant as your only option. Alcohol dependency, which affects ten per cent of men and four per cent of women in the UK, is a specific diagnosis in which the body has become dependent on alcohol. If you stop drinking you get delirium tremens, hallucinations and potentially life-threatening withdrawal symptoms. It is the cause of 33,000 deaths in the UK every year. Problem drinking, however, can mean anything from teenagers who get into fights after a few pints, to couples guzzling wine at home in the evening. Don't wait for a wake-up call, such as needing a drink in the morning to steady you, or missing work due to a hangover.

THE SCIENCE

The government-recommended two to three units per day for women and three to four for men is easy to exceed. Wine bars typically serve huge glasses that contain three or four units each, and some strong lagers can have over four units a pint. Many people assume that the government errs on the side of safety and they can get away with more, but research suggests that the UK guidelines are, if anything, a bit too liberal.

Excessive drinking adversely affects every organ of the body: it causes liver disease, gastritis,

can damage the pancreas, increase blood pressure and put you at risk of heart attack and stroke; it can raise your risk of diabetes and sexual dysfunction and make you more likely to get oral and stomach cancers and certain neurological diseases.

On top of that, alcohol irritates the gut wall, causing inflammation and meaning that you don't absorb nutrients from food so efficiently. In particular, it interferes with the uptake of folate, which helps to produce new cells, so if you drink a lot it's important to eat a diet rich in folate. Heavy

Eating well is good for our mental as well as our physical health, while eating badly will have long-term cumulative effects on virtually every aspect of our wellbeing. It's not just about getting the nutrients required for all the body's metabolic processes to be carried out; there's a social and a self-care aspect to healthy eating as well.

Many people live alone, work late and have busy social lives, which means they don't have the time to cook and eat well, and ready meals provide a convenient, if unhealthy, alternative. However, we also find that those with low self-esteem are less likely to eat well. As they tuck into their bland microwaved meals or chocolate biscuits, they are reinforcing the message that they are not worth taking any trouble over. If they could manage to cook and eat a delicious meal made from fresh ingredients, they would be taking a step towards valuing themselves more highly.

Those with very hectic, stressful lifestyles who grab food on the run tend to opt for fatty, sugary junk foods because that's what their raised cortisol levels make them crave. It's true there are times when we all need a quick bite to stave off hunger, but sitting down to a home-cooked meal at least once a day should be part of everyone's routine.

Some of the conditions covered in this section are psychological, while others are associated with neurological problems or malfunctions in the brain's neuro-transmitters. We bring you the latest findings on the ways in which nutrients can affect your brain, and it's worth giving the recommendations a try, but you should seek help as well. Your doctor will take mental health problems every bit as seriously as if you had a broken leg, and there is a range of solutions they may be able to prescribe.

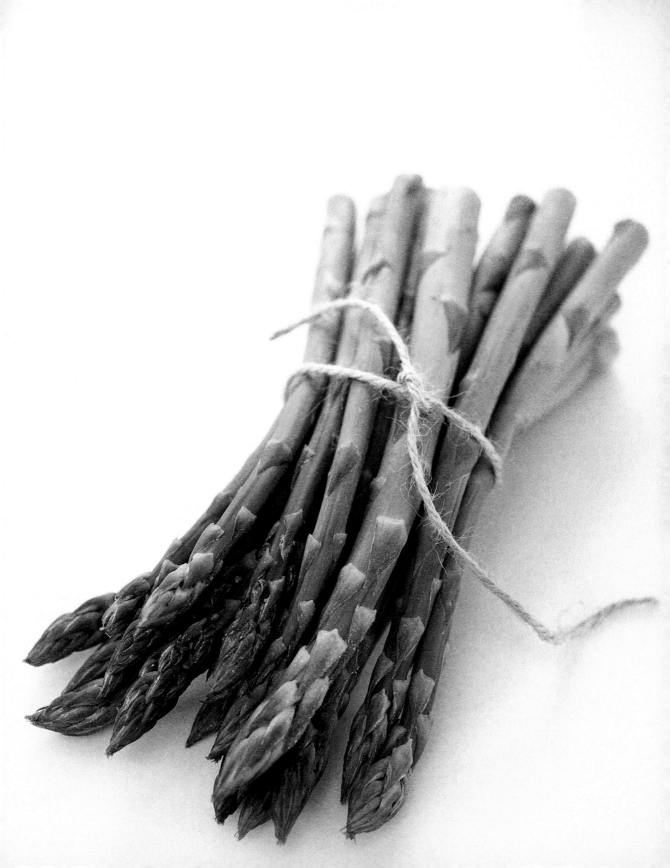

drinkers are likely to be deficient in a lot of the B vitamins, making them feel lethargic and lacking in energy. They can have a vitamin A deficiency, which is hard to make up because excess vitamin A is particularly toxic when you are drinking heavily, and they can also be calcium-deficient, putting them at risk of osteoporosis.

The good news is that if you stop drinking or cut back to well within the government guidelines before it's too late, you will be able to reverse most of the damage. But there's no way of knowing when that 'too late' will come, which is why you should reduce your drinking to healthy levels straight away.

Foods to Eat

- **Choose breakfast cereals that are fortified** with folate and iron, and other rich folate sources such as dark green leafy vegetables – spinach, kale and asparagus are all good.
- **Focus on foods containing B vitamins:** wholegrain bread and brown rice, milk and dairy produce, meat, fish, chicken and eggs.
- **Eat a wide range of different-coloured** fruits and vegetables for their antioxidants and fibre.
- **Stay well hydrated,** drinking at least two litres of plain water a day.

Foods to Avoid

- **Alcohol!**

Expert Tip

- **If you try to give up or cut down drinking** and then you relapse, don't despair. Most people need more than one attempt before finally getting there.

WARNING

If you are alcohol dependent, don't try to give up on your own. It's crucial that this is done under medical supervision.

CASE STUDY

Darren, a twenty-eight-year-old insurance broker, was brought in to A&E one night. He was found by the police sitting in the street, unable to speak clearly and partially unconscious. A toxicology screen showed he had taken alcohol only, no other drugs. He was given intravenous fluids to rehydrate him and blood tests showed that his liver enzymes were through the roof as a direct result of the mass of shots and beer he'd drunk. The raised liver enzymes showed his liver was inflamed – a clear case of alcoholic hepatitis. When he recovered enough to go home the next day he was informed of his blood test results and cautioned to watch his binge drinking because it was damaging his liver. He didn't think that he drank that much and argued that sometimes he didn't drink at all during the week. He didn't believe his blood tests could be accurate and, if they were, he doubted it was to do with his drinking. Darren is a classic example of someone with problem drinking.

ANOREXIA/BULIMIA

Eating disorders are extremely distressing to everyone involved – whether you're a sufferer or a friend or relative of one. It's vital that symptoms are picked up as soon as possible, so that medical and emotional help can be sought before the sufferer's health is permanently damaged. However, anorexics and bulimics will do their best to conceal the condition, making eating disorders hard to spot. Anorexics will be visibly thin, of course, but bulimics may have a normal body weight. Note that while both are most prevalent in women, lots of men are affected as well. Anorexics suffer from body dysmorphia, causing them to believe they are fat when they are, in fact, dangerously underweight. In severe cases they reduce their calorie intake until they are barely eating. Bulimics overeat or binge and then make themselves vomit and/or use laxatives in an attempt to purge themselves of the calories. Below you will find questions from two questionnaires that doctors use to diagnose eating disorders.

Do you ever make yourself sick because you feel uncomfortably full?

Do you worry that you have lost control over how much you eat?

Have you recently lost more than one stone in a three-month period?

Do you believe yourself to be fat when others say you are too thin?

Would you say that food dominates your life?[1]

Are you satisfied with your eating patterns?

Do you ever eat in secret?

Does your weight affect the way you feel about yourself?

Have any members of your family suffered with an eating disorder?

Do you currently suffer with or have you ever suffered in the past with an eating disorder?[2]

WARNING

Anorexia is not just a celebrity illness; it's a potentially life-threatening disease. It has the highest mortality rate of any psychiatric illness. That's why we are not going to offer quick-fix diet suggestions or 'cures'. If you think you have anorexia or bulimia, it is essential you get treatment from a qualified professional who can steer you on the path back to healthy eating.

The first step is admitting that you have a problem, and the second is seeking help for it. Don't think you can treat an eating disorder yourself: always get medical support.

1. *First five questions are from the SCOFF questionnaire, devised by researchers at St George's Hospital Medical School.*

2. *Second five questions are from the Eating disorder Screen for Primary care (ESP).*

ANXIETY

Anxiety is a normal reaction if a grizzly bear is walking towards you. In that circumstance, it's entirely appropriate. But if you frequently get anxious about perceived threats, to the extent that it interferes with your normal functioning, then you should seek help to deal with it. There are different types of anxiety: situational (for example, you feel anxious about speaking up in meetings at work), phobias (such as fear of heights, or spiders), post-traumatic stress disorder (after a terrifying experience) and generalized anxiety disorder (in which you have a pervasive sense of feeling anxious even when there are no specific triggers present). Anxiety can accompany depression, but it's also possible to be anxious without being depressed. Sometimes acute anxiety can cause panic attacks. These are severe, sudden-onset episodes in which sufferers get palpitations: they sweat, they feel nauseous and might throw up; they may faint, they get chest pains and some even fear they are going to die. It can be difficult to distinguish a panic attack from a heart attack because the adrenaline-related symptoms are similar.

THE SCIENCE

The first thing to do is reassure any anxiety sufferers that they are not going mad. Anxiety is a normal reaction, but in them it is becoming exaggerated and misplaced. Understanding what happens physically during a panic attack can help: for example, adrenaline causes your pulse to race and makes you sweat. Some of the symptoms are caused by hyperventilation, and one simple tip is to breathe in and out a paper bag. By reinhaling carbon dioxide you can help control hyperventilation. Understanding what is happening to you physically is one way of controlling the reaction.

Cognitive behaviour therapy is very effective for treating situational anxiety. In it, you will work through the triggers with a counsellor and figure out whether they are based on false premises. You will learn to take a step back and examine the thoughts that tend to be associated with your anxiety, because many people find this helps them to head off bouts of anxiety and panic attacks in future. Your counsellor may also teach you some relaxation techniques you can use to deal with anxious thoughts.

Your doctor might prescribe a short-term course of medication, and there are plenty of self-help techniques, including dietary ones.

Foods to Eat

- **Eat low-GL carbs and regular meals** and snacks to keep your blood sugar steady.
- **There have been promising results from trials** using magnesium supplements, but the jury is still out. However, including plenty of magnesium-rich foods in your diet, such as dairy products, fish, poultry, green vegetables, dried apricots and legumes, is a good idea.
- **The amino acids L-lysine and L-arginine** have been shown to help anxiety, and you'll find them in protein foods, such as fish, meat and poultry.

Foods to Avoid

- **Sugary foods and drinks** destabilize your blood sugar levels, which will affect your moods.
- **Alcohol and caffeine** are both mood destabilizers.

Expert Tips

- **Smoking can act as a depressant.** If you light up because you feel anxious, be aware that you will feel even worse an hour later when the blood nicotine levels drop again.
- **Regular exercise can help to combat anxiety** by promoting the release of serotonin, a hormone that improves mood.

CASE STUDY

Ruth, a thirty-five-year-old marketing rep, came to A&E with breathing difficulties and chest pain. She was terrified and thought she might have had a heart attack. She said she had been on a train when she suddenly started to sweat, got strong palpitations and felt sick and dizzy. While these symptoms can be a result of heart disease, she was tested and it was found this was not the case. It turned out that she had been treated for anxiety in the past and it had been getting worse again just before this. She was displaying the classic symptoms of a panic attack and was successfully treated with a short-term course of medication and cognitive behaviour therapy sessions.

See also: Depression, Cardiovascular disease

ATTENTION DEFICIT HYPERACTIVITY DISORDER

ADHD is a set of behavioural problems that make sufferers difficult to deal with. The symptoms include an inability to sustain attention or concentrate on the task at hand, restlessness, and a tendency to behave impulsively. An ADHD child won't be able to sit still for any length of time or maintain interest for long, even in a game that is fun, because they'll get up and wander off to explore the next thing that distracts them.

The disorder is thought to affect around two per cent of adults and between three and nine per cent of children of school age, although the symptoms can sometimes be confused with normal childish exuberance. It tends to be more common in boys than in girls, and is usually diagnosed between the ages of three and seven. For a diagnosis to be made, the behaviour should have continued for more than six months and be significantly affecting the sufferer's quality of life, in terms of their ability to make friends, thrive at school and even feed and dress themselves.

THE SCIENCE

The causes of ADHD are not clear, but it is known that there is less neurotransmitter activity in the parts of the brain that control attention levels. There appears to be a genetic link, and women who smoke during pregnancy are more likely to have children with ADHD. Exposure to lead (on old pipes or paintwork), and consumption of food additives and preservatives may contribute, as may watching a lot of television at a young age. There are loads of theories but no firm evidence.

There isn't a cure for ADHD but medication can help, and therapy might also be prescribed. It is important to provide a structured environment for ADHD sufferers, and that means regular mealtimes and a fixed bedtime. Children with ADHD may have low self-esteem so need lots of affection – which can be hard to provide when they are behaving disruptively! You might be able to identify and avoid triggers for bad behaviour, such as a situation where there are likely to be crowds of people, noise and bright lights. Your GP should be able to provide support in the form of health visitors, paediatricians or psychologists, as required.

A comprehensive overview of studies on ADHD and nutrition came up with one startling fact in particular: removing artificial food colours from the diet is thirty to fifty per cent as effective in improving behaviour and attention span as taking medication, and it doesn't have any side effects. This is the first thing to try if you or your child suffers from ADHD.

Some adult sufferers think that intolerances to wheat, nuts or dairy products can aggravate symptoms, so it might be worth keeping a food diary and excluding these one at a time to see if it makes a difference. Exclude each for four weeks, then reintroduce it before deciding whether to omit it long-term. Remember that if you do exclude dairy products long-term, you will need to make sure you get enough calcium from other sources. Only exclude dairy from a child's diet under the supervision of a qualified dietitian.

Foods to Eat

- **A varied diet** of fresh whole foods, using the Eatwell Plate as a model.
- **Include omega 3s in the diet** in whatever way you can. The salmon fish fingers overleaf are a good way to get a child to eat oily fish.

Foods to Avoid

- **Artificial food colourings and additives,** especially sunset yellow (E110), quinoline yellow (E104), carmoisine (E122), allura red (E129), tartrazine (E102) and ponceau 4R (E124). You'll find these in soft drinks, sweets, ice cream, cakes and biscuits and a number of other foods, so if buying packaged goods, read the labels carefully.
- **Sugar and caffeine in excess** can aggravate symptoms.
- **Adults can try excluding** wheat, nuts and dairy, one by one.

Expert Tips

- **If you are the parent of an ADHD sufferer,** don't blame yourself and try not to get angry with your child for behaviour they can't help. You'll learn to judge when they are being consciously naughty.
- **You may find there are local support groups** for ADHD sufferers. It's always good to know you're not alone.

WARNING

Anyone who takes medication for ADHD should have regular check-ups with their doctor to monitor them for side effects.

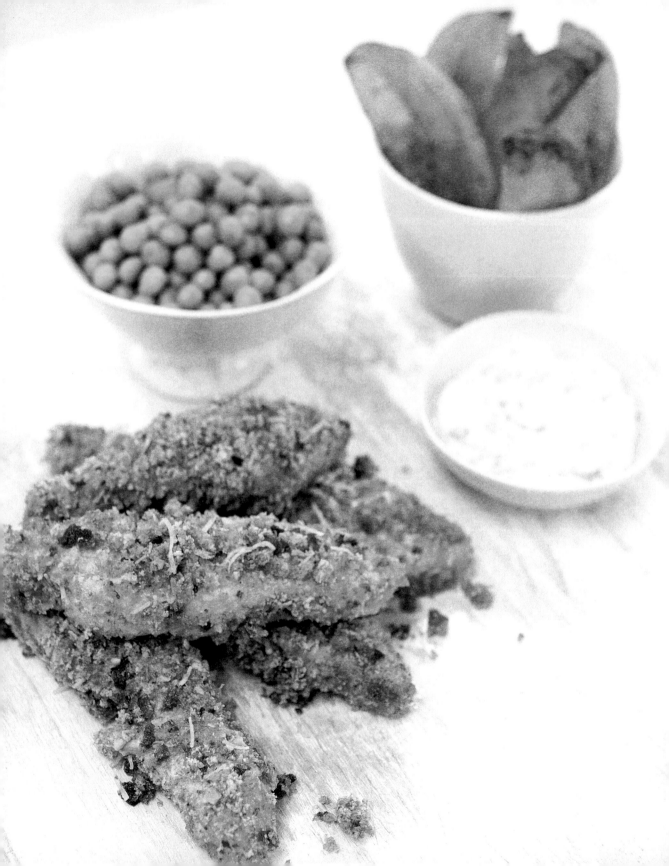

SALMON FISH FINGERS WITH A MINTY YOGHURT DIP, POTATO WEDGES AND PEAS

Serves 4 children
Preparation time: 20 minutes
Cooking time: 35 minutes

Ingredients

1. Preheat oven to 200°C/180°C fan/gas 6.

2. Slice the unpeeled potatoes into wedges. In a large bowl toss the wedges in the oil and paprika, arrange in a single layer on a pre-heated baking sheet and bake for 30 to 35 minutes or until the wedges are tender and golden.

3. Line a baking sheet with foil and spray with a little sunflower oil. Slice the salmon into fingers. In a large shallow dish combine the breadcrumbs and parmesan and, in another dish, whisk the eggs.

4. Take a finger of salmon and coat in the beaten egg, then roll it in the breadcrumbs and repeat the process once more. Continue to do this with all the fingers of salmon, making sure they are well and evenly coated in breadcrumbs. Place the fingers on the baking sheet and spray each one with a little more of the sunflower oil. Bake in the oven for 12 to 15 minutes or until crisp and turning golden.

5. Meanwhile, stir together the yoghurt, mint and sugar. Season with a little freshly ground black pepper. Serve the fish fingers with the yoghurt, wedges and peas.

The fish fingers can be made in a large batch and frozen.

For the Wedges

4 medium potatoes, scrubbed
1 tablespoon sunflower oil
½ teaspoon mild paprika

For the Fish Fingers

500g skinless salmon fillet
170g seeded wholemeal bread, blitzed into fine breadcrumbs
1 tablespoon finely grated parmesan
3 medium eggs
Sunflower oil spray
Freshly ground black pepper

To Serve

4 tablespoons Greek yoghurt
1 tablespoon mint leaves, finely chopped
Pinch of sugar
320g peas

Per serving: 627 kcals	43g protein	26g fat	5.5g saturated fat	60g carbs	5g sugar	11g fibre	0.8g salt

AUTISM

Autism is an umbrella term covering a wide spectrum of different behaviours and developmental problems. It's become a more common diagnosis over the last twenty years or so, but that doesn't necessarily mean it's more prevalent. It could just be that in the past, autistic children were labelled 'backward' or 'slow' or 'difficult'. Receiving this diagnosis for yourself or your child must be very distressing, but it's well worth knowing, because there is a lot that can be done to help sufferers.

Symptoms of autism include social and language delay, poor eye contact and a lack of empathy for other people's feelings. Sufferers often appear not to respond to questions, have trouble maintaining a conversation and resist physical affection. There may also be repetitive physical behaviours, such as rocking and foot tapping. Asperger's is a type of autism, but with milder symptoms than classic autism disorder. There is a wide range of severity, so that some people with autism lead relatively normal, independent lives, while others will always need care.

THE SCIENCE

There could be a genetic link in autism, and certain other factors may play a part as well: couples are more likely to have an autistic child if the mother smoked or was in contact with rubella during pregnancy, or if the father was over forty years old. The mechanism is not understood, but in brain scans it is apparent that the connections aren't working properly between the cerebral cortex, where sensory information is processed, language is developed and problems are solved, and the limbic system, which is responsible for emotional reactions.

If your child is not babbling and cooing, waving and pointing by the age of one, you should discuss it with your health visitor or GP, as it could be an early sign of autism. By the age of two, you would expect your child to be taking an interest in other children, bringing objects to show you and using their imaginations during play. If they are not doing this, your GP will probably refer you to a specialist, where there are physical and skills tests that can confirm a diagnosis.

There is no cure for autism, but there are structured programmes that can help an autistic child to develop social and language skills. They may thrive in creative environments where they can try music therapy and sensory therapy, for example. For adults diagnosed with autism, there is a range of care available, depending on what they need: sheltered housing, speech and language therapy, and in the UK they may be entitled to disability living allowance.

There have been dozens of studies of the effects of nutrition on autism, and some of the results look very interesting. In particular, excluding gluten (in wheat) and casein (in milk products) from the diet does appear to help symptoms in some sufferers, and the theory is that it's because of their effect on peptide molecules in the body. But the problem is that children with autism can be very picky eaters. It's quite common for them to eat only around twenty foods, and if fifteen of these contain gluten you can't really cut it out entirely. Any such changes should only be made with the support of a dietitian to ensure that the diet remains nutritionally sound.

Foods to Eat

- **A trial in which B6 and magnesium supplements** were given to autism sufferers proved inconclusive, but it may be a good idea to make sure you include plenty of foods containing them in your diet: eggs, whole grains, brown rice, yeast, dried apricots, nuts and dark chocolate.

- **Omega 3 oils may be helpful,** so include a serving of oily fish every week, or focus on other sources such as nuts and seeds.

- **A ketogenic diet** (high-fat, adequate protein and low-carb) may improve symptoms in autistic children, but what we don't yet know is the long-term effects of feeding them a diet that is high in fat. There's a lack of data so far, and this must be followed under guidance of a specialist. For more about this kind of diet, see under Epilepsy (page 236).

Foods to Avoid

- **You could try excluding casein** (found in milk products) and gluetin (found in wheat) but only under the supervision of a dietitian.

Expert Tips

- **Some alternative therapists suggest** treating autism with a process called chelation, in which you swallow infusions designed to expel toxins such as heavy metals from the body. The majority of clinicians and scientists think this is a complete scam and should be avoided.

- **Reports that the MMR vaccine can cause autism** were discovered to be completely unfounded.

WARNING

It can be hard caring for someone with autism, so do get all the support you can. See the National Autistic Society website www.autism.org.uk for more advice.

CHRONIC FATIGUE SYNDROME

The causes of Chronic Fatigue Syndrome, also known as ME, are not well understood. If you are constantly exhausted, your doctor will first refer you for tests to rule out other possible causes such as anaemia, diabetes, thyroid problems, sleep apnoea or lupus. Sometimes, you can feel exhausted for several months following a viral infection, or it could simply be that you are not sleeping well. Once all other possible causes have been ruled out, your doctor might consider CFS if you have the kind of tiredness that is not relieved by taking a holiday, but he or she may avoid using the term because it's a bit of a negative label to carry. However, the good news is that most people's symptoms improve over time and some make a full recovery.

THE SCIENCE

Some researchers think that CFS is triggered after a bout of glandular fever, from which the immune system doesn't fully recover, but it also frequently occurs after a traumatic life event such as bereavement or divorce. Poor diet, stress and lack of exercise might be further contributory factors. In around a third of sufferers, CFS is associated with depression, and it can also occur at the same time as fibromyalgia, a condition which causes pain in the muscles and joints throughout the body.

If you are diagnosed with CFS, it's a good idea to find out as much as you can about the condition, and take control over your symptoms rather than letting them control you. Around a third of sufferers benefit from taking antidepressants and most of those with mild to moderate symptoms find that regular, low-impact aerobic exercise improves their condition over the long term. You might start with a ten-minute walk twice a week, and try to build up to swimming, cycling or another exercise of your choice for thirty minutes three times a week. Experiment and structure your days to maximize your energy, but try to resist the temptation to nap during the day, as this could mean you don't sleep so well at night. Establish a restful evening routine, and make sure your bedroom is dark and cool so that you get good-quality sleep.

There have been lots of interesting studies on nutrition and CFS. We've summarized the most convincing findings below. The most important thing is to eat a varied, healthy diet with lots of fruit and veg, fish and whole grains.

- **In a randomized, controlled trial,** 45g of eighty-five-per-cent-cocoa dark chocolate per day was found to be very effective in reducing fatigue, anxiety and depression and restoring energy levels. The bonus is that the trial subjects didn't experience any weight gain so this is definitely worth trying (see recipe on page 117).

- **A small pilot study found that drinking a bottle of yoghurt drink** with probiotic lactobacillus casei shirota every day helped ease symptoms of anxiety in CFS sufferers compared to the control group.

- **Get a good intake of omega 3 oils** from salmon, sardines, herring, mackerel, trout – the dark-skinned fish are best – as well as flaxseeds, walnuts and olive oil.

- **Monosodium glutamate** (a thickener and flavour enhancer used in Chinese food) may make CFS symptoms worse. When eating in Chinese restaurants, be wary of anything with a sauce: opt instead for steamed fish with ginger and spring onions, or crispy duck.

- **Aspartame, an artificial sweetener found widely** in diet foods such as low-fat yoghurts, low-sugar drinks, cereals, ice-creams, meal replacements and chewing gum, is best avoided if you suffer from CFS.

- **Anecdotal evidence suggests** that acupuncture can help with CFS symptoms.

- **Don't be tempted to try lots of herbal preparations.** It's understandable that you want to try anything you can to find a cure but there are some potent compounds out there that haven't been through rigorous medical testing.

- **Cognitive behaviour therapy can be very useful,** and some areas have clinics offering a wealth of advice for chronic fatigue sufferers.

WARNING

Don't self-diagnose CFS. You must go to a doctor and get tested to make sure your fatigue isn't the result of some other condition.

See also: Anxiety, Depression, Fibromyalgia, Insomnia

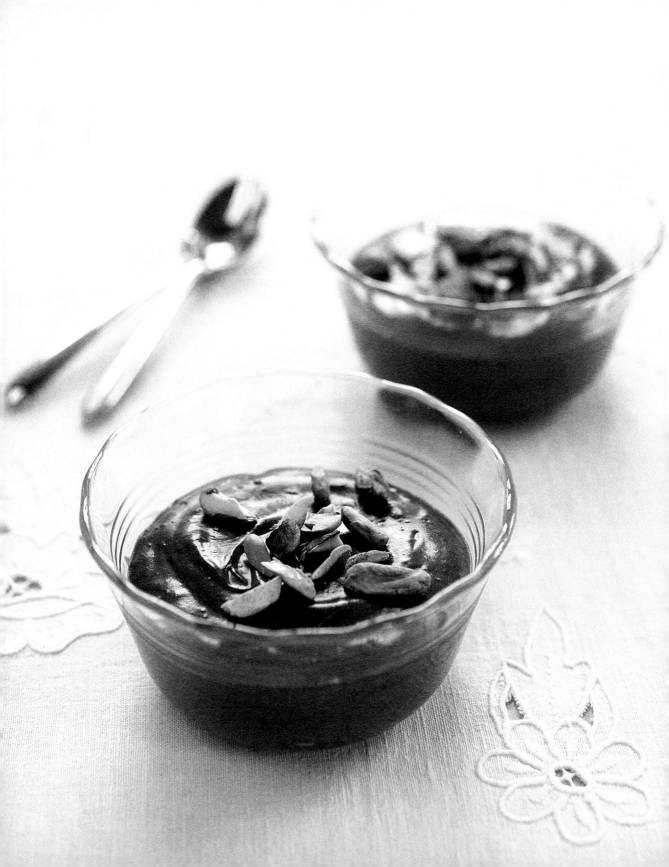

CHOCOLATE, ORANGE AND PISTACHIO MOUSSE

Makes 2
Preparation time: 10 minutes + 1 hour cooling time

1. Break the chocolate into pieces and put into a bowl with the orange zest, over, but not touching, a pan of simmering water. When the chocolate begins to melt, turn the heat off. Once the chocolate has fully melted, remove the bowl from the pan to cool a little until it is warm rather than hot.

2. Separate the eggs. Whisk the egg whites into soft peaks, add the sugar, and whisk briefly.

3. Stir the egg yolks into the melted chocolate and then whisk in a spoonful of the egg white. Gently fold the rest of the whites into the chocolate mixture until just combined. Spoon into 2 small glasses and chill for 1 hour.

4. To serve, spoon some yoghurt on top of the mousse, if liked, and scatter over some pistachio nuts.

Ingredients

60g 85 per cent dark chocolate
Finely grated zest of 1 unwaxed orange
2 medium eggs
2 teaspoons caster sugar

To Serve

100g Probiotic natural yoghurt, optional
1 tablespoon unsalted pistachio nuts, roughly chopped

Per serving: 343 kcals | 13g protein | 20g fat | 8g saturated fat | 30g carbs | 27g sugar | 2g fibre | 0.3g salt

DEMENTIA/ ALZHEIMER'S

Dementia is a deterioration in cognitive function. It affects memory and the ability to make decisions and judgements. An early sign might be someone repeating an anecdote they have already told you, or frequently being unable to remember a name. There are different kinds of dementia, with different physical causes. In Alzheimer's disease (accounting for around sixty per cent of dementia cases), plaques grow around brain cells and disrupt the normal function. In vascular dementia, not enough blood is reaching the brain cells because of arterial blockages; it is associated with high blood pressure and high cholesterol. In Lewy body dementia, there are cellular changes in the brain. If you suspect someone may have a form of dementia, it can be awkward to bring the subject up, but it's important to get a diagnosis as early as possible, because there are medications that can slow the progress of this cruel disease.

THE SCIENCE

A GP will probably take some blood tests to rule out other possible causes of forgetfulness, such as vitamin B deficiency. It can be useful if a close friend or relative attends the appointment with the patient, who may not be aware of the extent of their own memory loss. Memory and cognitive tests, such as the Mini Mental State Examination, may be given, and then the patient might be referred for a CT scan to see what is going on in the brain. Typically, dementia occurs in people over the age of sixty-five, but it is possible to have early-onset Alzheimer's. You are more likely to suffer from dementia if there is a family history. People with Down's Syndrome are more likely to get it, as are those who have high blood pressure, high cholesterol or Parkinson's disease. The sad fact is that dementia is progressive, but a new generation of anti-cholinesterase inhibitor drugs can increase the blood flow to the brain's neurotransmitters and help with memory function and concentration. Not everyone can take them and there are some side effects, but they are well worth a try, especially in the early stages.

Smoking increases the risk of developing dementia, because it promotes thickening of the arteries and poor blood supply to the brain. Long-term heavy drinking can also be a cause, as can obesity, lack of exercise and eating a high-fat diet, because all of these promote atherosclerosis, or clogging up of the arteries. Everyone over the age of fifty should have their blood pressure and blood cholesterol checked regularly to ensure they remain within safe limits. Dementia can also be associated with raised levels of homocysteine in the blood. Normally, you break down homocysteine naturally with the help of B vitamins and folic acid, but if you have B vitamin deficiency, this mechanism can fail. For dementia prevention, focus on a diet that has plenty of folate and vitamin B12, get regular exercise and keep yourself at a healthy weight. Vitamin D deficiency has also been linked to Alzheimer's, so get regular short intervals of sun exposure. There are ongoing trials into the effectiveness of high-strength vitamin B supplements in the treatment of Alzheimer's, and while there aren't any definitive conclusions yet, you could try taking vitamin B supplements (up to the recommended daily allowance) if you have been diagnosed with the disease. Check with your specialist first.

Turmeric contains curcumin, which has antioxidant, anti-inflammatory and anti-plaque agents.

Eat plenty of B-vitamin-containing foods: whole grains, beans, eggs, fish, organ meats and green leafy vegetables. After diagnosis, ask your specialist about taking high-strength vitamin B supplements.

Vitamin D is found in dairy, eggs and fatty fish.

Eat plenty of omega 3s: oily fish, nuts, seeds and avocados. In one study on mice, these reduced the growth of plaques by seventy per cent.

Foods to Avoid

Saturated fats, which can lead to arterial blockages.

Excessive alcohol also leads to clogged arteries.

Foods to Eat

A diet rich in polyphenols, such as blueberries (see recipe on page 121), pomegranates, red grapes, green tea, cranberries and red wine (one glass a day) may suppress the onset of dementia by scavenging free radicals and preventing oxidative damage to the brain.

Expert Tips

It's important to stay active and keep up a range of interests in old age. Get as much exercise as you can, and maintain a social life.

Partners and relatives of dementia sufferers should let them remain as independent as possible for as long as possible, within safe limits.

CASE STUDY

A t the age of sixty-eight, George still works on his own fruit and veg stall. His son insisted that he consulted his GP after noticing that George was having trouble calculating change for customers. Tests confirmed early dementia and also found that his blood pressure and blood cholesterol were far too high. He modified his diet and started taking an anti-cholinesterase drug to manage his condition. A few months later, his family report there have been marked improvements in his memory.

WARNING

You may be able to continue driving for some time after a dementia diagnosis, so long as you are not putting other road users at risk, but it is a legal requirement that you inform the DVLA.

See also: High blood pressure, High blood cholesterol, Diabetes, Parkinson's disease.

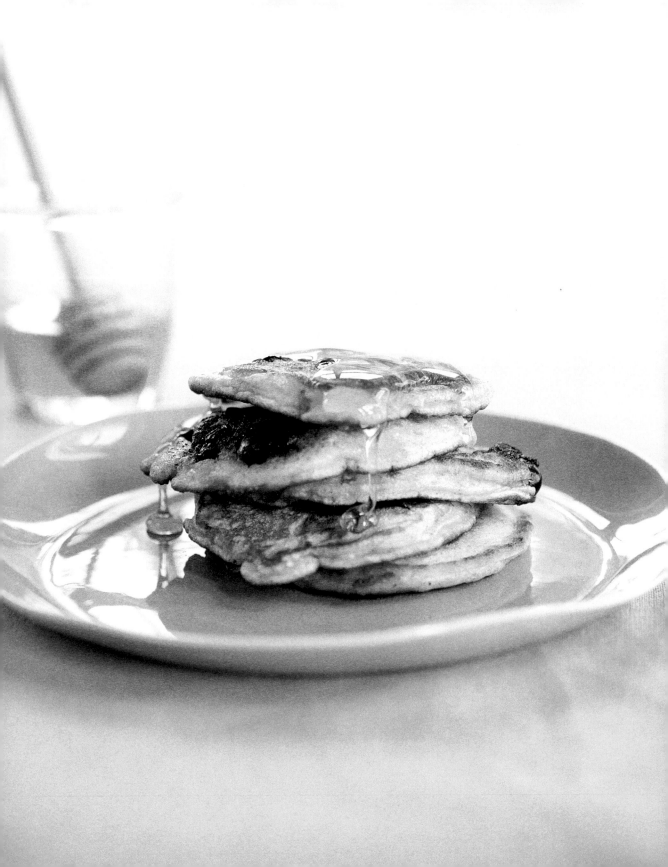

BLUEBERRY BUTTERMILK PANCAKES

Serves 4
Preparation time: 10 minutes
Cooking time: 20 minutes

Ingredients

Sift together the two flours, baking powder, bicarbonate of soda, salt and sugar in a large bowl.

Whisk together the eggs, buttermilk and milk. Make a well in the dry ingredients and pour in the egg mixture, then whisk the wet into the dry.

Heat a large frying pan over a medium heat, wipe the pan with a little sunflower oil, spoon a small ladleful of the batter into the pan and sprinkle over some blueberries. Repeat with 2 to 3 more, depending on the size of your pan; the pancakes should be about 8 to 10cm in diameter. When the mixture starts to bubble on the surface, carefully turn over and cook on the other side; depending on your pan this should take about 2 to 3 minutes on each side. Repeat until you have used all of the batter.

Serve warm.

These would be extra delicious served with low-fat probiotic natural yoghurt and a drizzle of either maple syrup or honey.

100g wholegrain flour
100g plain flour
½ teaspoon baking powder
½ teaspoon bicarbonate of soda
Pinch of salt
2 tablespoons caster sugar
2 medium eggs
125ml buttermilk
250ml semi-skimmed milk
250g blueberries
1 tablespoon sunflower oil

| Per serving 317 kcals | 13g protein | 8g fat | 1g saturated fat | 51g carbs | 16g sugar | 6.5g fibre | 0.9g salt |

DEPRESSION

There are circumstances in which depression is completely normal. If you are bereaved or your partner leaves you, it is appropriate to be depressed. However, if that depression drags on for months or years, during which you are unable to function properly at work or in your social life, you need to do something about it. Anyone who has suicidal thoughts should find someone sympathetic to talk to as soon as possible: a friend, a doctor, a qualified counsellor or, preferably, all three.

THE SCIENCE

There are many situations that can trigger depression: postnatal after having a baby; bipolar, which is characterized by periods of depression followed by periods of a very high mood and manic behaviour; seasonal affective disorder (SAD), caused by lack of light in winter; grief after bereavement; and chronic depression, which just won't shift. There can be physical as well as psychological symptoms: lack of energy, sleep disruption, slow speech and movement, change in appetite, constipation, and changes to the menstrual cycle.

At least one in ten people will get depression at some stage in their lives (and by this, we don't just mean they will feel a bit down for a week or so; they will have a serious depression that lasts for several weeks or months). In some cases it is triggered by a stressful life event; yet more become depressed after they are diagnosed with a serious illness; and alcohol, smoking and drugs can all cause depression.

Depending on the severity of your depression, your GP might prescribe antidepressants, counselling or a combination of the two, but there is lots of lifestyle advice that can help as well. For mild to moderate depression, a cardiovascular exercise programme is strongly recommended; try to get at least thirty minutes, three times a week, and make sure you get out of breath to benefit from the release of endorphins, the brain's natural feel-good hormones. For SAD, there are effective treatments involving light therapy, in which you sit for about twenty minutes a day in front of a lightbox emitting light at a similar frequency to sunlight. And all types of depression can be eased by eating a healthy diet and taking good care of yourself physically. If you feel low, focusing on looking after your physical health is a good start on the road back to psychological health.

Foods to Eat

- **There's been strong evidence that omega 3 fatty acids can help to relieve depression,** so increase your intake of oily fish to two or three portions a week (see recipe on page 124), and add some avocados, nuts and seeds to your diet. Use olive or rapeseed oil for cooking and dressing salads.

- **Folate, vitamin B12 and magnesium deficiencies have all been linked to depression,** so get plenty of whole grains, pulses, dairy products, eggs, organ meats, nuts, dried apricots and dark chocolate.

A Mediterranean diet is a great way to combat depression. The herb oregano can boost serotonin levels.

Foods to Avoid

According to one study, aspartame, the artificial sweetener found in low-sugar diet products such as fizzy drinks, yoghurts and chewing gum, seems to make symptoms worse in a lot of people suffering from depression. However, this was strongly refuted by the manufacturer and a later study found no adverse reactions. You could try avoiding aspartame to see if it makes a difference for you but read food labels carefully, because it crops up in a surprising range of products.

Alcohol is a depressant. It's the last thing you need if you're already depressed.

Expert Tip

No matter how much you might feel like shutting the door on the world, try to stay socially active. Joining some kind of therapy group and discussing your problems with others could make a difference.

WARNING

If you have suicidal thoughts, or if you are self-harming, do seek help. Don't give up hope, because there's a lot that can be done to make you feel better.

See also: Anxiety, Insomnia

TROUT STUFFED WITH ALMONDS, SPINACH AND MUSHROOMS

Serves 4
Preparation time: 15 minutes
Cooking time: 20 minutes

1. Preheat oven to 180°C/160°C fan/gas 4.

2. Heat the oil in a frying pan over a medium heat and add the onion and garlic, cook for 3 minutes or until just tender. Add the mushrooms and cook for a further 3 to 4 minutes. Add the spinach to the pan and stir until just wilted. Remove from the heat and add the herbs, breadcrumbs and almonds, season with plenty of freshly ground black pepper, and set aside to cool.

3. Evenly fill each fish with the stuffing, securing with a couple of cocktail sticks. Place the fish on a baking tray lined with foil and sprayed with olive oil spray. Place the trout in the oven and cook for 10 to 12 minutes.

4. While the trout are cooking, steam the asparagus and broccoli for 4 to 5 minutes until al dente. Serve with the trout.

Ingredients

4 brown or rainbow trout, gutted and cleaned
Olive oil spray

For the Stuffing
1 tablespoon olive oil
1 small onion, finely chopped
1 garlic clove, peeled and crushed
100g chestnut mushrooms, chopped
75g baby leaf spinach, washed and dried
1 tablespoon chopped mint
1 tablespoon chopped parsley
2 tablespoons wholemeal breadcrumbs
75g flaked almonds
Freshly ground black pepper

To Serve
150g asparagus, trimmed
150g tender stem broccoli

Per serving: 404 kcals | 47g protein | 23g fat | 1.5g saturated fat | 4g carbs | 3g sugar | 3g fibre | 0.4g salt

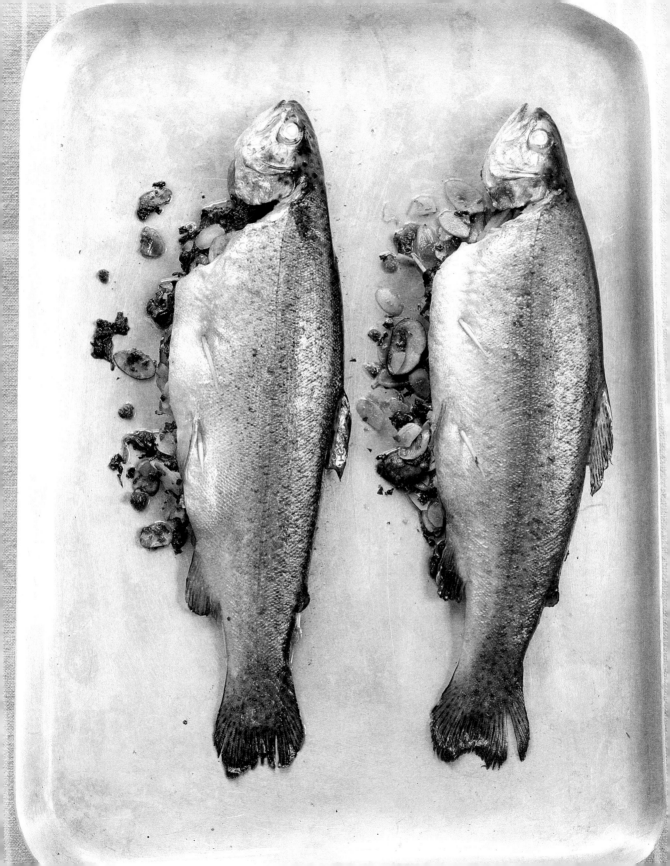

FIBROMYALGIA

Fibromyalgia is a condition in which sufferers feel pain throughout their body, particularly in the back and neck, but elsewhere as well. It gets better or worse depending on external triggers such as hot weather, stress levels and the amount of restful sleep that has been possible, but it is a chronic condition that sufferers need to learn to manage; there is no cure.

THE SCIENCE

No one knows what causes fibromyalgia. One theory is that there is a problem with the neurotransmitters signalling pain to the brain, making sufferers more sensitive to pain. The condition sometimes seems to have been triggered after a traumatic event, and it can co-exist with depression, anxiety, chronic fatigue syndrome and irritable bowel syndrome. Treatments might include painkillers, antidepressants or anti-inflammatory medication, but lifestyle modifications are essential. A muscle-strengthening exercise regime can help a lot, but you may need to ask a physiotherapist to devise routines that you can follow without exacerbating your existing muscle and joint pain.

There has been a lot of research into how nutrition can help, and it has been found that quite a restrictive vegetarian or vegan diet relieved symptoms in the majority of sufferers. It might be hard to follow the strictest regimes all the time, but dietitians often advocate an 80/20 rule: follow the diet at least eighty per cent of the time.

Foods to Eat

- **A vegetarian diet may help fibromyalgia sufferers.** Studies have found that their brains are low in the amino acid tryptophan, and it's possible this could have been caused by a diet high in animal proteins.

- **A small trial in which fibromyalgia sufferers** ate a low-salt, raw food, vegan diet showed a marked decrease in pain levels, but it could be difficult to stick to this long-term.

- **Fibromyalgia sufferers need a good intake of omega 3 oils** from oily fish, nuts, seeds or avocados.

Foods to Avoid

- **Fibromyalgia sufferers should avoid saturated fats as far as possible,** both in animal foods and those containing palm oil and coconut oil.

- **Some people think that aspartame** (artificial sweetener) and MSG (a thickener in many sauces, particularly in Chinese food) make fibromyalgia worse.

- **It might be worth keeping a food diary** and excluding certain foods which have been found to trigger fibromyalgia symptoms: wheat, dairy, citrus fruits, corn and sugar. Exclude them one by one, for at least four weeks each.

See also: Anxiety, Arthritis, Chronic Fatigue Syndrome, Depression, Irritable Bowel Syndrome

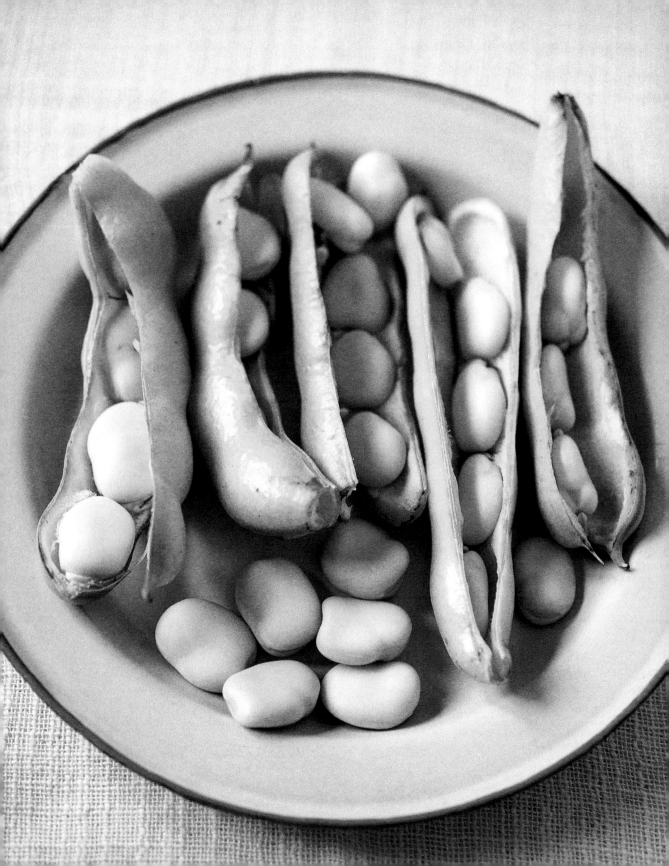

DEEP SOUTH
RICE AND BEANS

Serves 4
Preparation time: 15 minutes
Cooking time: 40 minutes

1. Cook the rice as per pack instructions.

2. Once the rice is cooked, heat the olive oil in a large frying pan or casserole dish, tip in the mushrooms, peppers and onion, fry for 4 to 5 minutes over a medium to high heat. Stir in the Cajun spices, add the chilli and tomatoes and heat through.

3. Stir in the cooked rice along with the kidney beans, lentils and herbs, then cook gently for 2 to 3 minutes to heat the beans and lentils through. Season to taste with the salt and freshly ground black pepper. Serve garnished with a few basil leaves.

Ingredients

200g easy-cook wholegrain brown rice
4 tablespoons olive oil
6 chestnut mushrooms, chopped
1 green pepper, deseeded and sliced
1 red pepper, deseeded and sliced
1 large onion, finely chopped
1 tablespoon Cajun spice mix
1 small green chilli, deseeded and finely chopped
3 tomatoes, chopped
1 x 215g tin red kidney beans, rinsed and drained
125g ready-to-eat puy lentils
1 tablespoon chopped fresh basil
2 tablespoons fresh thyme, leaves only
Salt and freshly ground black pepper
Basil leaves, to garnish

Per serving: 351 kcals	9g protein	13g fat	2g saturated fat	52g carbs	6.5g sugar	8g fibre	0.3g salt

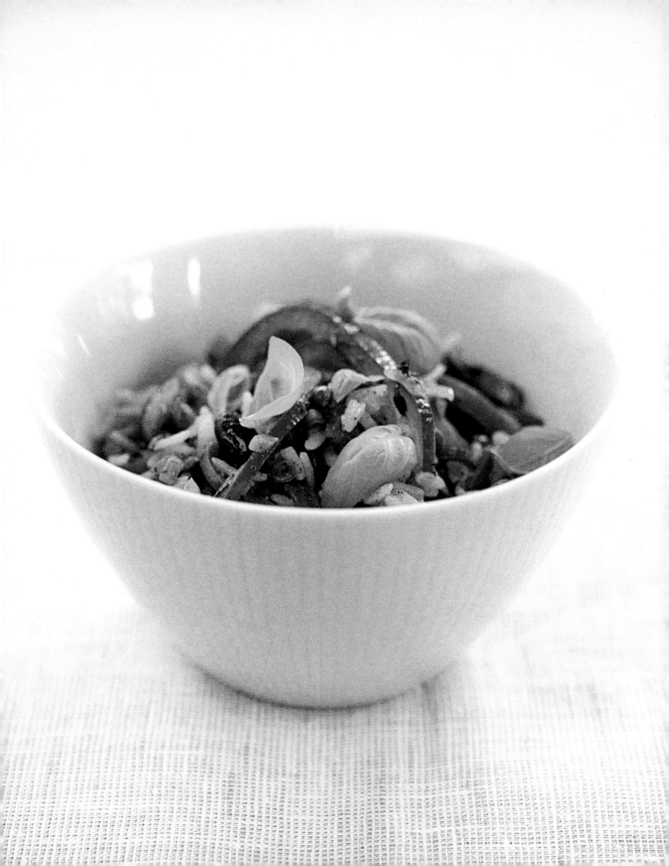

INSOMNIA

We all have nights when we toss and turn, unable to nod off: There are dozens of possible causes: stress, anxiety about a forthcoming event, jet lag, hormone swings, overindulgence in food, caffeine or alcohol, smoking cigarettes, or it can be a side effect of some prescription medications. You could be wakening up due to a condition such as restless legs or not getting refreshing sleep because of snoring – your own or your partner's! And there are several medical conditions that can make it difficult to get a full night's sleep.

If you are finding that you regularly fail to get enough sleep, start keeping a sleep diary, in which you note down the time you went to bed, how long it took to get to sleep, the number of times you woke in the night and any naps you took during the day, as well as the times at which you ate meals, your alcohol consumption and the exercise you took. Once you've kept this for a couple of weeks, take it to your GP and between you, you may be able to detect what's causing the problem and come up with a solution. You might be referred for tests to rule out certain conditions, but don't assume that you will automatically be given a prescription for sleeping pills; they tend to be seen as a last resort, or are only used in the short term (seven to ten days) to cut you some slack.

THE SCIENCE

For restful sleep, the bedroom should be cool and dark, without the distraction of streetlamps shining through the curtains or winking lights on computer consoles. When it's dark, your brain secretes more melatonin, a hormone that plays a critical role in our sleep patterns. Medical advice is to avoid caffeine, smoking and alcohol for six hours before you go to bed, avoid exercising within four hours of going to bed, and avoid eating a heavy evening meal. Establish a bedtime routine that helps you to relax, perhaps having a bath or reading a book rather than watching a violent thriller on TV. Try to go to bed around the same time every night, get up at a reasonable hour in the morning and avoid napping during the day if you can.

If you don't find relief from following those tips, your GP might refer you for some kind of counselling, in which you may be taught relaxation techniques and other ways to help you wind down at night. What you eat and drink in the hours before bedtime is particularly important, though.

Foods to Eat

- **Have a high-carb bedtime snack.** This stimulates the release of insulin, which can help an amino acid called tryptophan to cross the blood/brain barrier and create melatonin. Choose something low-GL, such as porridge or a couple of oatcakes.
- **Alternatively, turkey is a good source of tryptophan,** so you could try eating a couple of slices. Beef, ham, eggs, anchovies and quorn are also good, or you could have a handful of mixed seeds or soy beans.

- **Night-time milk** – from cows that have been milked at night – contains high levels of melatonin that can help you sleep.
- **Make sure you eat enough magnesium-rich foods** – bananas, dried apricots, avocados, almonds, cashews, peas and beans – as insomnia can be a symptom of magnesium deficiency.
- **Chamomile and passion flower tea** can aid restful sleep (or try the recipe on page 133).
- **One study suggests** two servings of tart cherry juice may help regulate sleep.

Foods to Avoid

- **One standard alcoholic drink probably won't make a difference,** but excess alcohol decreases the REM sleep we all need and disrupts the body's natural rhythms. The more you drink, the worse the disruption.
- **The elderly can be particularly sensitive to caffeine** as their systems are slower at clearing it from the blood. They should address their caffeine intake, whether it's from tea, coffee, cola, chocolate or over-the-counter medications such as paracetamol.

Expert Tips

- **Get some form of exercise every day,** even if it's just walking briskly to the shops. But make sure you do it more than four hours before bedtime.
- **Avoid television or computer** use just before bed.

WARNING

Sleeping pills should only be used for short periods, and you should take the lowest possible dose, as it is easy to become dependent on them.

See also: Restless legs, Snoring, Stress

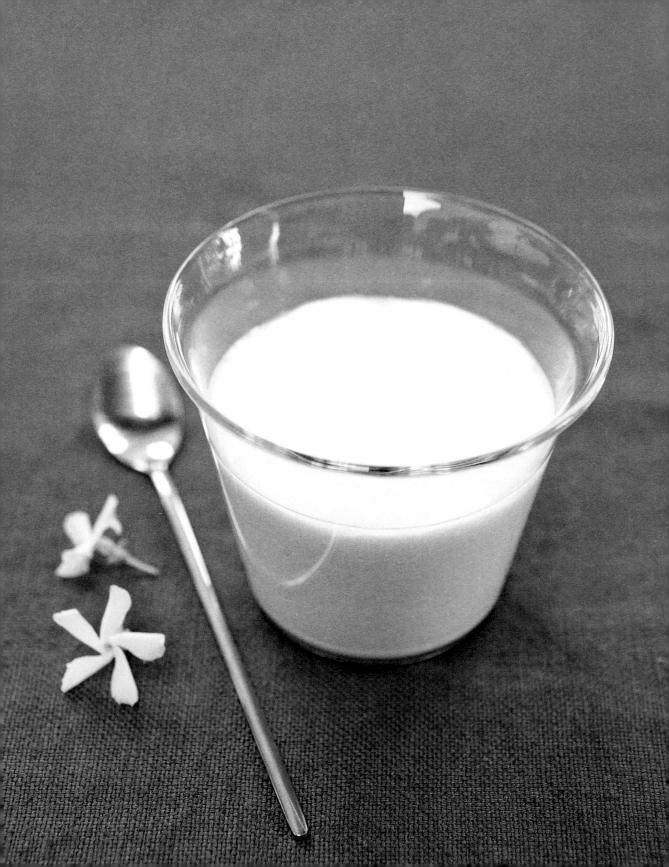

CREAMY CAMOMILE FOOL

Serves 2
Preparation time: 25 minutes + 1 hour chilling

Ingredients

1. Pour the boiling water over the tea bag and sugar, stir to dissolve the sugar and leave to infuse for 20 minutes.

2. Gently fold together the crème fraîche, yoghurt and lemon zest. Gradually fold in the camomile water. Spoon into glasses and chill for 1 hour. Serve.

1 camomile tea bag
3 tablespoons boiling water
2 tablespoons caster sugar
200g low-fat crème fraîche
100g low-fat vanilla yoghurt
Finely grated zest of 1 lemon

Per serving: 250 kcals	5g protein	16g fat	10g saturated fat	24g carbs	22g sugar	0g fibre	0.02g salt

SMOKING ADDICTION

Health warnings are plastered all over cigarette packs in stark black and white letters, so we don't need to reiterate the detail here. But we're going to anyway. The basic truth is that fifty per cent of all smokers in the UK die prematurely because of their smoking, and the remainder who make it into old age are likely to have far more health problems than their non-smoking friends. Are you in denial about the extent of your smoking? Realize that harm is being done whether you smoke forty cigarettes a day or one small cigar a week, and the whole body is affected. Smoking causes or increases the risk of the following: Cancers of the lung, mouth, throat, larynx (voice box), oesophagus, cervix, prostate, pancreas, bladder and kidney. Circulatory diseases such as heart attack, heart failure, arterial disease, claudication of the legs causing pain due to furred-up arteries, angina, stroke, aneurysm, raised blood pressure and impotence. Lung diseases such as emphysema (when the lungs can't inflate properly), pneumonia, bronchitis and asthma. Gastrointestinal problems such as Crohn's disease, gum disease, heartburn and ulcers. Various other symptoms such as reduced fertility, premature skin ageing, and loss of taste and smell.

THE SCIENCE

When you light a cigarette, nicotine droplets are absorbed through the soft tissues of the mouth and throat, causing the release of adrenaline, the hormone we normally release when stressed. Your heart rate rises by as much as thirty per cent, the blood supply is diverted away from the skin and intestine, and carbon monoxide replaces oxygen in the lungs. These heightened responses begin to decrease within an hour or so after finishing the cigarette, and your body starts to crave the next one. The relief they feel on lighting a cigarette makes many smokers think it helps them to deal with stress, but in fact it is smoking that causes the feelings of stress in the first place by triggering the release of adrenaline. Smoking also causes the release of dopamine in the brain, making us feel good so that we seek out the same effect again – but note that dopamine is also released in response to healthy behaviours, such as eating a good meal or having good sex, so you don't need a cigarette to benefit.

The good news is that when you give up, your body will gradually return to normal, so long as you haven't already incurred any lasting damage. Within forty-eight hours, the nicotine will be out of your system and your skin pallor should improve. Three to nine months after giving up, your lung function will have improved significantly. After five years, your risk of heart attack is almost as low as that of a non-smoker and after ten years, your risk of lung cancer is half that of a smoker.

Don't despair if you don't manage to quit on the first attempt; the majority of smokers have two failed attempts before finally getting there. Do approach your doctor, because you are more likely to succeed with the help of nicotine replacement therapies, prescription drugs such as Champix, counselling, acupuncture, hypnotherapy or support groups.

Smokers have a higher requirement for vitamins and minerals than non-smokers because of the oxidative effects of smoking on the system, but this doesn't mean they should take supplements. Antioxidants taken in supplement form, particularly vitamins A and E, can become pro-oxidant and increase the cancer risk in smokers.

Smoking is an appetite suppressant, so many people do tend to gain some weight when they give up, but why not use it as an opportunity to address your diet and adopt a healthier eating pattern? Focus on eating well, don't worry about putting on the odd pound or two, and you will regain good health more quickly.

Foods to Eat

- **Smokers are particularly deficient in vitamin C,** so they need to make sure they get a wide range of fruits and vegetables in their diet: rich sources of vitamin C include citrus fruits, strawberries, kiwis, broccoli, cabbage and Brussels sprouts.
- **When you give up, eat regular, small meals** and snacks that are rich in low-GL foods to keep blood sugar steady, and drink plenty of water to flush out the nicotine.

Foods to Avoid

- **Vitamin and mineral supplements,** especially those containing vitamins A and E.

Expert Tips

- **Save the money you don't spend on cigarettes** to buy a treat, such as a family holiday. If you currently smoke twenty a day, you could save £2500 in a year of not smoking.
- **Beware of passive smoking:** the smoke coming from the sides of a burning cigarette is actually more dangerous than the stuff that smokers inhale.

WARNING

See also: Cancer, Cardiovascular disease, Stroke, High blood pressure, High cholesterol, Asthma, Crohn's disease, Receding gums, Indigestion.

STRESS

A short burst of stress can give us the push we need to do our best in an exam, or to run away from a dangerous situation. But long-term stress has debilitating effects right throughout the body and can cause a wide range of symptoms you might not realize are associated with it: depression, food cravings, irritable bowel syndrome, loss of appetite, chest pains, dizziness, erectile dysfunction, loss of sex drive, excess sweating, insomnia, weight gain and difficulty concentrating. Then there are the things you don't even notice it's doing, such as suppressing the immune system and raising blood pressure and cholesterol levels, which can lead to heart attacks and strokes. It might require some major readjustment of your priorities in life, but it's essential for your health to get stress under control. 'Type A' personalities were first described in the 1970s: competitive, driven and hard-working, these are people who experience a lot of stress and, independent of other factors, they have a higher risk of having a heart attack than Type Bs or Cs.

THE SCIENCE

When we feel stressed, our bodies release the stress hormones adrenaline, noradrenaline and cortisol. These speed up the heart rate and divert blood to the muscles of the arms and legs, ready for sudden movement. They make us breathe faster to take in more oxygen. At the same time, kidney function slows, digestion slows and the liver releases fat and sugar into the bloodstream to provide energy. These reactions would all be very useful if we had to run away from an escaped tiger in a zoo, and in that situation the stress hormones would dissipate within a couple of hours after we reached a place of safety or the tiger was recaptured. But if the stressful situation continues long-term, there's a build-up of stress hormones in the bloodstream, which leads to many adverse effects on health.

The first thing to do about long-term stress is to learn to control your reaction to stressful events. Saying 'no' to a demanding boss or people who are behaving unreasonably is a great skill to learn. If you have money worries, seek help to address them. Consider getting counselling to deal with relationship or family problems, or anger management lessons to reduce feelings of rage. Find ways of relaxing that you enjoy, whether it be meditation, exercise or a favourite hobby. And try the following nutritional advice to help protect you from the worst effects of stress.

Foods to Eat

- **A low-GL approach that stabilizes blood sugar will help,** and you should eat small meals and snacks every three hours throughout the day (see recipe on page 138).
- **Lack of folate and the B vitamins thiamine, niacin and cobalamin** can contribute to feelings of exhaustion and negative mood. Make sure you eat plenty of whole grains, beans, meats, fish and poultry, avocados, broccoli, Brussels sprouts and asparagus.
- **Low levels of selenium** can contribute to low moods. For a concentrated source, nibble a few Brazil nuts every day.
- **Keep yourself well hydrated** with plenty of plain water.

Foods to Avoid

- **Cortisol can make us crave sugary, fatty foods,** but you should resist this craving because the sugar rush followed by the drop will exacerbate symptoms of stress.

- **Some people use caffeine** to help them get through the working day and alcohol to help them come down afterwards, but both of these cause the same physiological reactions as stress in the body and should be avoided.

Expert Tips

- **Aerobic exercise** (the kind that makes you out of breath) will help to dissipate stress hormones and promote the release of serotonin, which is a mood enhancer. Try to get at least three thirty-minute sessions per week, more if you can.
- **Smoking is one of the worst things** you can do for your stress levels. Giving up can be stressful in the short term, but it is essential for your long-term health.

WARNING

Long-term stress puts pressure on virtually every system in the body, and sooner or later something will give way as a result.

See also: Depression, Irritable Bowel Syndrome, Erectile dysfunction, Low sex drive, Insomnia, High blood pressure, High cholesterol.

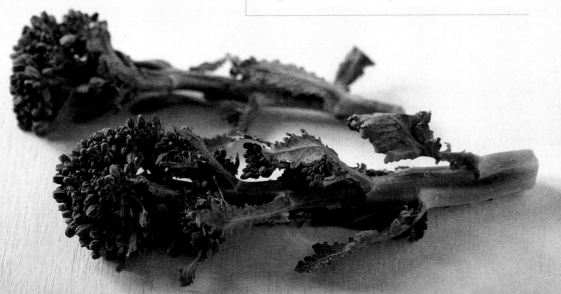

MIXED
SPICED NUTS

Cooking time: 30 minutes

1. Preheat the oven to 100°C/80°C fan/gas ¼.
   Line a large baking sheet with greaseproof paper.

2. Heat a large heavy-based frying pan over a medium
   heat. Tip in the almonds, cashews and salt, toast
   for 1 to 2 minutes, tossing the nuts around the pan.
   Add the soya beans and pumpkin seeds to the
   pan, drizzle in the oil and cook the nuts, stirring
   frequently until lightly golden. Sprinkle the paprika,
   cayenne and freshly ground black pepper into the
   pan and continue to cook for 1 minute.

3. Stir the honey into the nuts and toss well to coat.
   Cook for a further 1 to 2 minutes or until the honey
   starts to caramelize, then remove the pan from the
   heat. Tip the nuts on to the baking sheet and place
   in the oven for 20 to 30 minutes.

4. Remove the nuts from the oven and leave to cool
   completely to room temperature. Store the cooled
   nuts in an airtight jar or tin. Serve as nibbles or
   have as an on the go snack.

Ingredients

200g blanched almonds
200g unsalted cashews
½ teaspoon salt
200g dried soya beans
200g pumpkin seeds
2 tablespoons olive oil
2 teaspoons smoked paprika
1 teaspoon cayenne pepper
Freshly ground black pepper
1 tablespoon runny honey

| Total: 4503 kcals | 198g protein | 358g fat | 50g saturated fat | 127g carbs | 44g sugar | 64g fibre | 0.27g salt |

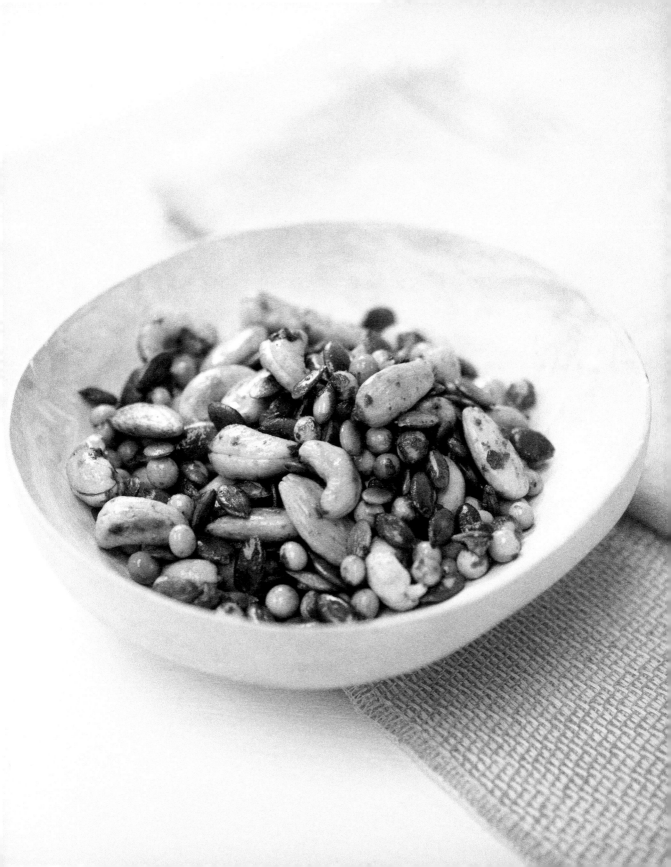

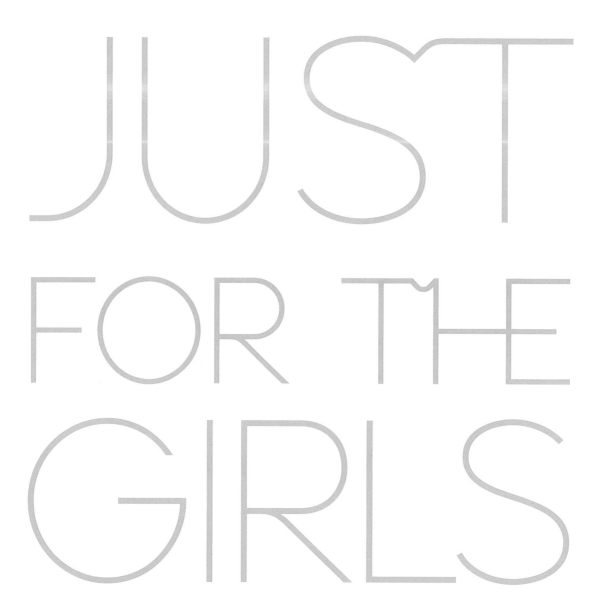

JUST
FOR THE
GIRLS

Throughout women's lifetimes, their hormones shift and change: as they reach puberty, enter their childbearing years and perhaps become pregnant, breastfeed, experience peri-menopause and then enter menopause itself. The intricate dove-tailing of hormones is a delicate operation, and very easily affected by external factors, such as women's weight, stress levels, exercise and sleep patterns, medication they may be taking, lifestyle factors, such as alcohol and caffeine consumption and smoking, and, of course, their diets. It's not surprising that many conditions affecting women involve their hormones, which can lead to long-term health consequences if left untreated.

Drinking low levels of alcohol, avoiding saturated and transfats in the diet, and keeping refined foods (with preservatives, colourings and other chemicals) to a minimum can help to achieve all-round good health, as can eating plenty of good-quality proteins and lots of fresh fruits and vegetables. In particular, omega oils are important in maintaining the balance of women's hormones as they move through the various stages of their lives; not only do they reduce an inflammatory process that may underlie some of the health conditions affecting women, but the omega 3 oils affect the way that oestrogen is handled in the body.

What we eat most definitely affects the way we feel, and the complex balance of our hormones. While we can't control the process of ageing, we can control the way we feel and the symptoms that accompany it. Food is one of the best ways to do this.

ENDOMETRIOSIS

Endometriosis occurs when the lining of the womb (the endometrium) becomes displaced and grows on other organs outside the womb (most commonly the ovaries, fallopian tubes and the tissues holding the womb in place). Every month, the tissues in your womb thicken before your period, and if you don't become pregnant, they break down and leave the body as blood. Endometrial tissue that is growing elsewhere in your body goes through the same process, but because there is no way for the blood to escape, you may experience pain, swelling and scarring that can lead to fertility problems. You might experience no symptoms, or you may have lots: chronic pelvic pain, pain during sex, changes to your period (including irregular bleeding or heavy periods), painful bowel movements, fatigue and swelling of your lower abdomen. Diagnosis is normally made by the nature of your symptoms, and can be confirmed by *laparascopy*.

THE SCIENCE

The cause of endometriosis is still unclear, but we do know that it is more common in women who have never had a baby, and it often appears in your early twenties. There is also some family history of this condition, so if your mother or sister suffers, you are more likely to have it as well. Treatment normally involves taking hormones (such as the oral contraceptive pill) to try to regulate your cycle – or manipulate it so that you don't experience symptoms. Surgery is another option, and it would be designed to remove the patches of endometrial tissue in your pelvis. Another solution might be a hysterectomy (removing your womb completely), which while not for everybody can be a relief for some women.

Foods to Eat

- **A plant-based diet can make a huge difference;** one study found that women who eat more than thirteen servings of green vegetables every week have a seventy per cent lower risk of endometriosis than women who eat fewer than six.

- **Plenty of omega 3 oils,** found in nuts, seeds and oily fish (such as salmon, mackerel, trout) can act as a natural anti-inflammatory to ease symptoms. Walnuts appear to be particularly effective.

- **Peas, beans, pulses, red and purple berries, garlic, apples, nuts and seeds, carrots and rhubarb contain natural phytoestrogens,** which can block oestrogen receptors, thus balancing hormones (see recipe on page 145).

- **You may be more at risk of anaemia** if you regularly experience heavy bleeding, so increase your intake of iron-rich foods (such as leafy green vegetables and dried fruit) and see your doctor if you are unusually pale or tired.

- **A low-GL diet** has shown to help reduce painful symptoms

- **Green tea may help** to reduce endometrial growth

Foods to Avoid

- **Red meat, ham and processed meats** such as bacon may increase your risk of endometriosis.

- **Saturated fats,** such as butter and fatty meats, refined sugars and honey can cause inflammation.

- **Caffeine increases oestrogen levels** (endometriosis is an 'oestrogen sensitive' condition), and also causes abdominal cramping.

- **Soya contains a chemical that seems to be problematic for some women with endometriosis;** although it is a phytoestrogen, it is particularly powerful and not appropriate for sufferers.

- **Refined and processed foods that contain additives,** preservatives and other 'E' numbers can put pressure on your liver, which is responsible for processing hormones.

Expert Tips

- **Evening primrose oil and vitamin B6** (found in fortified cereals, baked potatoes, bananas, chicken, pork, beef, trout and avocado) may help to relieve symptoms such as pain and heavy bleeding around the time of your period. Both are available in supplement form and can be taken daily. It can take a couple of months to see any improvement.

- **Get plenty of regular exercise,** which can reduce your risk of endometriosis by seventy-five per cent. Thirty minutes, three or four times a week, is advisable.

- **Try to maintain a healthy weight;** fat can produce oestrogen and make the condition worse.

WARNING

Always report any abnormal bleeding to your doctor, and make sure your cervical smears are up to date.

See also: Heavy, painful periods, Anaemia

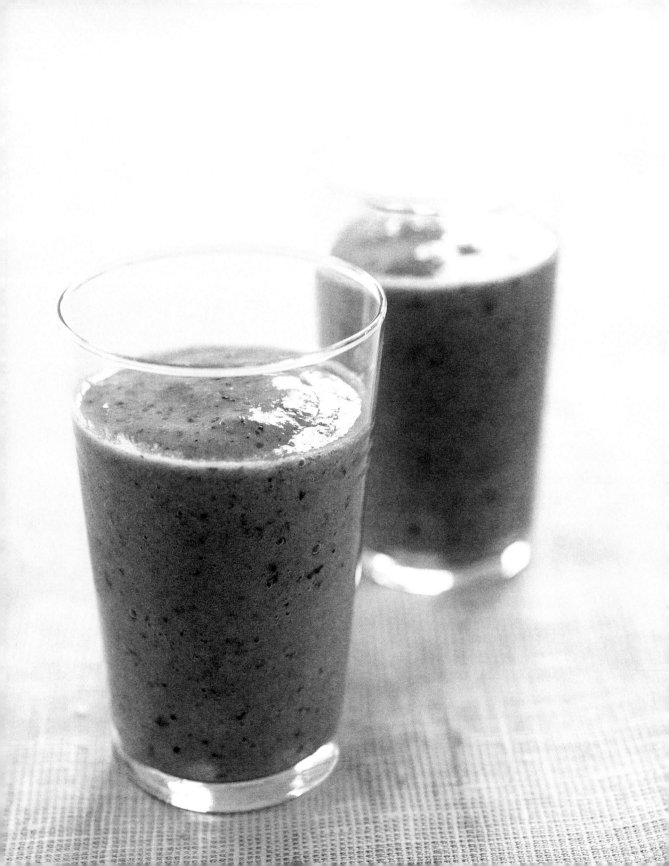

BERRY SUPER SMOOTHIE

Serves 2
Preparation time: 5 minutes

Ingredients

The trick is to start with the fruit and add the spinach to taste – not allow the smoothie to taste of spinach!

1. Tip the fruit into a jug blender and add a splash of the milk, then blend until smooth. Gradually add the remaining milk.

2. Add half of the spinach and blend, have a taste and, if liked, gradually add the remaining spinach – you shouldn't be able to taste the spinach! Depending on the sweetness of the fruit you may need to add a little honey to taste. Serve immediately.

1 banana, peeled
150g fresh or frozen blueberries
100g fresh or frozen raspberries
400ml skimmed or semi-skimmed milk
50g baby leaf spinach
1 teaspoon honey, optional

Per serving: 161 kcals | 9.5g protein | 1.1g fat | 0.5g saturated fat | 30g carbs | 27g sugar | 6g fibre | 0.3g salt

HEAVY, PAINFUL PERIODS

Heavy periods *(menorrhagia)* are diagnosed when an unusually high amount of blood is lost across several consecutive periods. They can occur on their own, or in combination with other symptoms, such as menstrual pain (known as dysmenorrhoea). Blood loss is considered to be excessive if you need to change your pad or tampon every hour for at least two or three hours in a row, pass large clots, experience 'flooding' through to clothing or bedding, or have periods that last longer than five to seven days. Cramping, lower back pain and nausea or changes in bowel habits can accompany heavy, painful periods. Diagnosis of conditions that may be at the root of the problem may include a vaginal examination, a *biopsy* of the lining of your womb, *blood tests* and/or a pelvic *ultrasound* or *transvaginal* scan.

THE SCIENCE

There are a number of health problems that can cause heavy and/or painful periods, and these include endometriosis, fibroids (small growths in the lining of your uterus), thyroid problems, the months leading up to the menopause or infections. Treatment would be based on the cause of your bleeding or pain. For example, if you suffer from fibroids, you may be treated with hormones, such as the birth control pill, which helps to even out your hormone cycle and reduce surges of oestrogen that can make things worse, or even a type of surgery to shrink fibroids. An IUD called the Mirena coil contains the hormone progesterone, which can help to thin the lining of your uterus and reduce symptoms.

Foods to Eat

- **A diet that is rich in plant foods,** such as nuts, seeds, pulses, fruit and vegetables, can help to reduce oestrogen, which can be at the root of the problem. In fact, one study found that a low-fat vegan diet reduced the duration and severity of pain in subjects. Fresh fruit and vegetables also contain vitamin C, which is required for your body to absorb iron from your food.

- **Increase your intake of oily fish,** which contains omega 3 oils that can reduce the inflammation causing pain.

- **Eat foods rich in zinc** (such as oysters, wheat germ, peanuts, sesame and pumpkin seeds, beef and cocoa). Zinc is vital for a healthy reproductive system and hormone balance.

- **Wholegrains and pulses are rich in vitamin B,** which can reduce unusual blood clotting and inflammation (see recipe on page 148).

Foods to Avoid

- **Red meat and other foods high in saturated fat** can cause inflammation that makes the problem worse; however, if you do cut red meat from your diet, make sure that you get plenty of other iron-rich foods (see page 217 and 277), or try to eat meat once a week. Heavy bleeding can put you at an increased risk of anaemia.

- **Tea and coffee can prevent the absorption of iron,** which can lead to anaemia. The caffeine they contain may also raise your oestrogen levels and make symptoms worse.

- **Alcohol puts pressure on your liver,** which is responsible for converting excess oestrogen into weaker forms; avoid it completely if you have heavy, painful periods.

- **Unless you are menopausal, avoid soya,** which can raise oestrogen levels to a point that symptoms become worse.

Expert Tips

- **There is some evidence that taking vitamin B1 in supplement** form can be effective in reducing pain. Try 100mg per day to see if there is any improvement.

- **Keep a record of your menstrual cycles and any other bleeding,** as well as the number of pads or tampons you are using. Write down any other symptoms, too. This will give your doctor a clearer idea of what you are experiencing.

- **Regular exercise can help with pain,** as it releases endorphins (feel-good chemicals); however, overly intense or long exercise sessions can exacerbate the problem.

WARNING

Contact your doctor if your bleeding has been heavy for more than three cycles, if you have a fever or abnormal discharge (smelly or thick, for example), if you experience bleeding or spotting between periods or after the menopause, if your pain is debilitating, if your bleeding lasts longer than a week or if it occurs between periods. Keep your cervical smear tests up to date.

See also: Polycystic ovaries, Endometriosis, Thyroid problems.

CASE STUDY

ucy was devastated by having to miss work for three days every month because of her heavy periods. People thought she was work shy, but she actually really enjoyed her job! What they didn't realize was that she would get floods of blood during the day, which regular tampons and towels just wouldn't hold back – something she found acutely embarrassing. The pain made her unable to concentrate and paracetamol or ibuprofen didn't help much. She reluctantly went to her GP, worried that she would be accused of over-reacting. Fortunately, this didn't happen. She underwent a cervical smear examination, which was reassuringly normal. Her doctor arranged a pelvic ultrasound scan and this showed a number of fibroids. After discussions with her doctor about the options, she ended up using a Mirena coil, which helped to reduce her bleeding and balance her hormones. She changed her diet to include far more fresh fruits and vegetables, and cut out coffee and alcohol completely. After just two months, her symptoms had almost completely disappeared.

ALMOND BREAKFAST MUESLI

Serves 8-10
Preparation time: 5 minutes
Cooking time: 30 minutes

1. Preheat the oven to 160°C/140°C fan/gas 3.

2. Stir together all of the ingredients for the muesli in a large bowl, spread on to a large baking tray and place in the oven for 25 to 30 minutes until golden brown, stirring half way through.

3. Leave to cool completely before storing in an airtight jar.

4. Serve with either yoghurt or milk and a mixture of berries and banana.

As well as being a wonderful breakfast, you could stir some muesli into a crumble topping.

Ingredients

100ml apple juice
1 tablespoon sunflower oil
100g flaked almonds
4 tablespoons sunflower seeds
2 tablespoons pumpkin seeds
1 tablespoon milled linseed/flaxseed
1 tablespoon sesame seeds

To Serve

Low-fat yoghurt or milk
Mixture of fresh raspberries, blueberries, strawberries and banana

Per serving: 160–128 kcals | 5–4g protein | 14–11g fat | 1.5–1.2g saturated fat | 3.5–2.8g carbs | 2–1.6g sugar | 1–0.8g fibre | trace salt

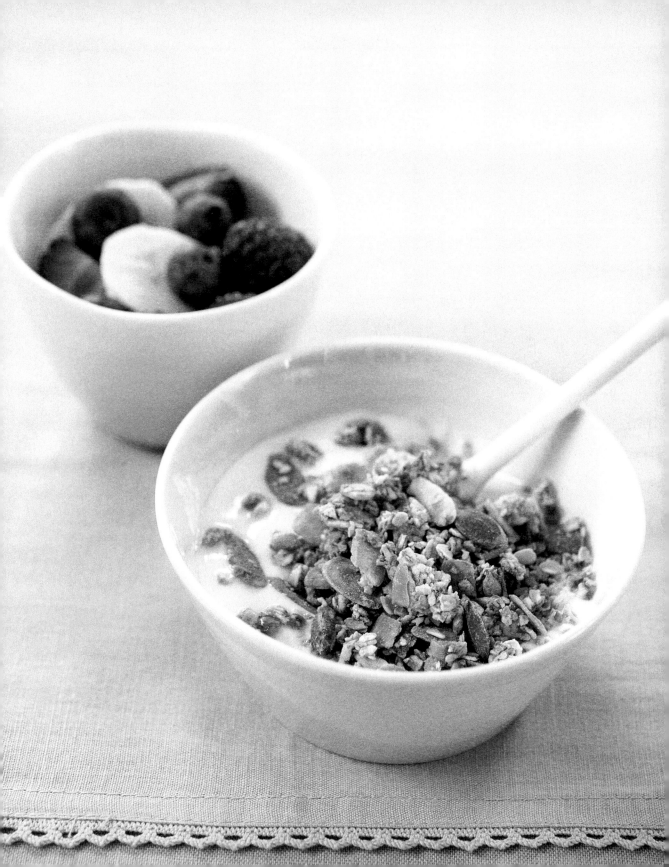

MENOPAUSE

Strictly speaking, menopause occurs when you have had no periods for twelve months. You will experience the most common symptoms of menopause, including hot flushes, night sweats, mood swings, memory problems, vaginal dryness, irregular periods and other issues, in the months or years before this, a time known as 'peri-menopause'. Menopause usually occurs around the age of fifty, but you can experience symptoms for years before this. Menopause is normally diagnosed by your symptoms and age; however, a blood test can be arranged to check your hormone levels to confirm the diagnosis.

THE SCIENCE

As we get older, the ovaries start to fail and less oestrogen is released. When this happens, the brain tries to jump-start the ovaries by releasing something known as FSH (follicle-stimulating hormone) and LH (luteinizing hormone) and it's these hormones, as well as the sputtering surges and troughs of oestrogen production, that cause symptoms. In a nutshell, irregular hormone patterns are to blame. Low doses of hormones are often prescribed (in the form of HRT), but this isn't always suitable (for example, if you have a history of breast cancer or if there's breast cancer in your family), and will usually only be prescribed short term. There are risks to taking HRT, such as increased risk of cardiovascular disease, that should be weighed up alongside the benefits.

Foods to Eat

- **Soya (in the form of soya milk, edamame beans or protein, for example)** can help to reduce the increased risk of cardiovascular disease and lowers the risk of osteoporosis, which can increase when oestrogen levels fall. It may help reduce the severity and frequency of hot flushes (see recipe on page 153).

- **Calcium-rich foods** such as leafy green vegetables, dried apricots, almonds and dairy produce will not only protect your bones, but also balance your moods.

- **Increase your intake of other phytoestrogens,** including flaxseeds and pumpkin, sesame and sunflower seeds, which help to keep hormones in balance.

- **Low-GL food and, in particular, whole grains,** will help to maintain steady blood sugar levels and ease mood swings; they are also rich in B vitamins which affect hormonal balance in your body and your mood (by raising serotonin levels).

- **Omega 3 oils,** found in flaxseeds, quinoa and oily fish, are anti-inflammatory, and can help to reduce a number of symptoms, such as hot flushes. They also help to protect your heart.

- **Plenty of fruit and vegetables,** which contain B vitamins (required for hormonal balance) and a host of other nutrients, including antioxidants, which can help to ease the process of ageing.

- **Vitamin E-rich foods** (such as sunflower seeds, almonds, peanuts, pine nuts, cooked spinach, avocado and dried apricots) have been shown to control and even eliminate hot flushes, and can also help with vaginal dryness.

Foods to Avoid

- **Spicy foods, caffeine and alcohol dilate the blood vessels,** and can make night sweats and hot flushes worse. Hot drinks may also exacerbate these symptoms. Alcohol puts pressure on your liver, which makes it less effective at processing oestrogens in your body.
- **Sugary refined foods can exacerbate mood problems and even memory loss,** and cause fluctuations in your blood sugar as well as making you overweight.
- **High levels of saturated fat,** in full-fat dairy produce and meat, for example, can increase your risk of heart disease and cause weight gain that may be difficult to shift.
- **Fizzy drinks** can weaken your bones and trigger hot flushes and night sweats.

Expert Tips

- **Smoking can increase** hot flushes and long-term health risks.
- **Breathing exercises can encourage relaxation,** which can reduce hot flushes and emotional symptoms, and help to lift your mood.
- **Regular exercise** can keep your bones strong, improve your circulation (which can have an impact on hot flushes), lift your mood and help you to manage your weight.
- **Getting a good night's sleep** can ease symptoms and help you to feel more energetic and balanced; aim for eight to ten hours per night.
- **Achieve a balanced weight;** being overweight can increase the number and duration of hot flushes and night sweats.
- **Wear layers** to control your temperature more easily.

WARNING

Any changes in your menstrual cycle should be reported to your doctor to rule out any other problems, such as an underactive thyroid. Never assume that unusual or debilitating symptoms are normal; talk to your doctor to check that menopause, and not something else, is at the root.

See also: Osteoporosis, Heavy periods, Anxiety, Low sex drive, Headaches, Depression, Weight gain, Wrinkles

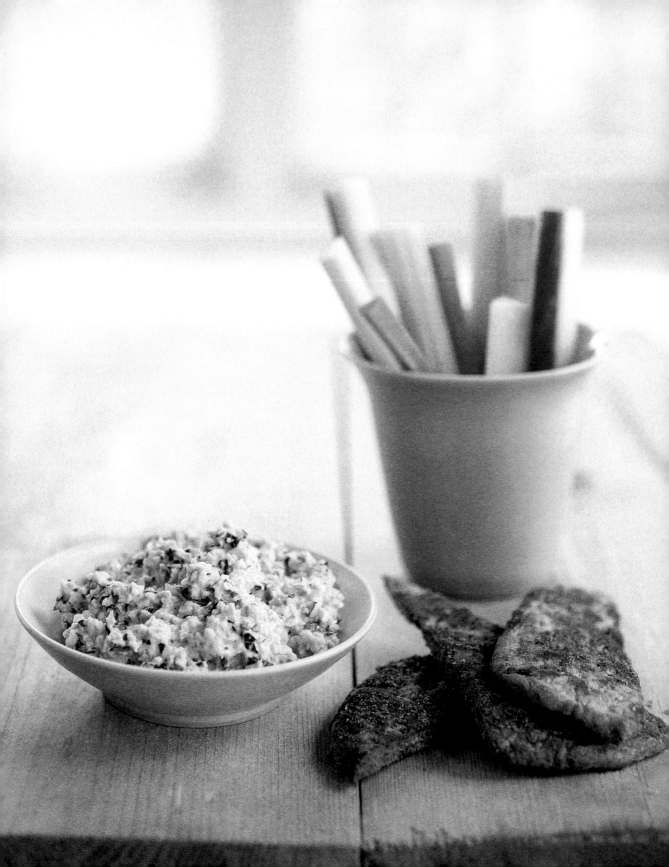

EDAMAME DIP WITH SPICED PITTA CHIPS AND CRUDITÉS

Serves 8 as a snack
Preparation time: 20 minutes
Cooking time: 5 minutes

1. Preheat the oven to 180°C/160°C fan/gas 4.

2. Slice the pitta breads into bite-sized wedges, mix the oil and spices together in a bowl and toss the pitta wedges in the mixture to coat. Spread the pitta on to a large baking sheet, then bake for 20 to 25 minutes or until crisp and golden.

3. Steam or blanch the edamame beans for 4 to 5 minutes until tender, run under cold water and drain. Tip into a food processor along with the remaining dip ingredients and blitz until smooth.

4. Serve the dip with the pitta chips and crudités.

Ingredients

For the Pitta Chips

4 wholegrain pitta breads
1 tablespoon olive oil
1 teaspoon ground cumin
1 teaspoon garlic powder
¼ teaspoon cayenne pepper

For the Dip

400g shelled edamame beans
200g silken tofu or fat-free yoghurt
2 tablespoons olive oil
Finely grated zest and juice of 1 lemon
2 cloves garlic, crushed
20g bunch mint, leaves only, roughly chopped
1 teaspoon ground cumin
Freshly ground black pepper

For the Crudités

2 carrots, peeled and cut into sticks
2 stalks celery, cut into sticks
¼ cucumber, cut into sticks

| Per serving: 230 kcals | 12g protein | 9g fat | 1g saturated fat | 25g carbs | 3g sugar | 5g fibre | 0.4g salt |

POLYCYSTIC OVARIES

Polycystic ovary syndrome (PCOS) is a condition in which the ovaries develop a number of harmless cysts around the edges. These cysts are follicles containing eggs which have not developed properly. Many women have cysts on their ovaries; however, in PCOS there are a number of additional symptoms, including irregular or very light periods, difficulty becoming pregnant (mainly because the follicles do not develop enough to release an egg), weight gain, skin problems (such as acne) and excessive hair growth – often on the face – but thinning hair or hair loss on the scalp. Not all women with PCOS experience symptoms, though. The condition is usually diagnosed when they are unable to get pregnant, if they have irregular periods or excessive hair growth. An *ultrasound* scan and *blood tests* can confirm the diagnosis.

THE SCIENCE

The causes of PCOS are not completely clear, but we do know that if you have a resistance to insulin (a hormone produced by your pancreas that controls your blood sugar), you will be more susceptible. In insulin resistance, your tissues become resistant to the effects of insulin, causing your body to produce more to compensate. High levels of insulin cause the ovaries to produce too much of the hormone testosterone, which affects normal ovulation and interferes with the development of your egg-producing follicles.

Hormonal imbalances are also a common culprit, and these can include higher-than-usual 'male' hormones (known as androgens), such as testosterone, LH (luteinizing hormone), which stimulates ovulation, and prolactin, which usually encourages the breast glands to produce milk in pregnancy. You may also have lower-than-usual thyroid hormones and progesterone.

Around twenty per cent of women have inconsequential cysts on their ovaries. PCOS affects about five per cent of women, and many of those are overweight or obese. Losing five per cent of your body weight is recommended but may be difficult as women with PCOS have a lower metabolism and increased levels of hunger hormone. A family history of PCOS, diabetes and high cholesterol will make you more at risk of this condition. Treatment will normally involve weight loss, hormone treatments and, rarely, surgery on the ovaries that may stimulate ovulation.

Foods to Eat

- **A low-GL diet is very important,** to keep your blood sugar levels stable and prevent spikes of insulin being produced. It can also improve your menstrual cycle and help you to lose weight, which is the primary treatment for PCOS.

- **Omega 3 oils,** found in oily fish and flaxseeds, for example, can help to reduce inflammation underpinning the condition.

- **Phytoestrogens,** such as soya, can help to balance hormones in the body.

- **Green tea and blueberries** both contain compounds that can discourage weight gain (particularly around your middle) and also enhance your metabolism.

- **Healthy proteins** (such as pulses, nuts, tofu, eggs, fish, chicken, meat and vegetarian meat substitutes), as well as healthy fats (such as those found in olives and avocados) are important to slow down the absorption of carbohydrates in your diet and keep your insulin levels low.

- **Walnuts and almonds** have been found to be particularly helpful in managing androgen levels.

- **Spearmint tea helps to reduce** androgens whilst cinnamon may help to stabilize blood glucose levels.

- **Eat plenty of fibre,** found in whole grains, pulses, fruit and vegetables, to slow down the digestion of sugar in the body, preventing spikes in insulin, and also reducing excess oestrogens in the body.

- **Chromium is an extremely important mineral** if you have PCOS. It helps to encourage the formation of glucose tolerance factor (GTF), which is a substance released by the liver that is required to make insulin more efficient. You can find it in meat, sweetcorn, sweet potato, apples, eggs and broccoli.

- **Eat vitamin B-rich foods,** which help to control weight, turn fat, sugar and protein into energy, control blood sugar and fat metabolism, and encourage the health of your liver to convert old hormones into harmless substances that can be excreted from your body. Whole grains, pulses, molasses and Marmite are good sources of B vitamins, as are many fruits and vegetables (see recipe on page 156).

Foods to Avoid

- **Avoiding high-GL carbohydrates** can help to keep your insulin levels down. Avoid white, refined carbohydrates and sugar wherever possible.

- **Cut out caffeine,** which can increase oestrogen levels.

- **Transfats and high levels of saturated fats can cause inflammation** and worsen insulin resistance, which seems to occur in many cases of PCOS.

- **Alcohol puts pressure on your liver,** making it less efficient at clearing away excess hormones.

- **Avoid low-carbohydrate diets** that are high in saturated fat; these are particularly dangerous for women with PCOS, who already have an increased risk of heart disease. Excess protein can also increase insulin production.

Expert Tips

- **Achieving and maintaining a healthy weight** is the very best way to address this condition.

- **Regular exercise can reduce high testosterone levels** and improve excess hair growth and insulin resistance.

- **Relax and reduce stress as much as possible.** Adrenaline is produced when we are under pressure and this hormone can make PCOS much worse.

WARNING

See your doctor if you suffer from PCOS and become pregnant, as you will have a higher risk of complications, such as pre-eclampsia.

If you are prescribed the drug Spirinocatone for PCOS you shouldn't take it if you are trying to get pregnant or are pregnant.

See also: Acne, Infertility, Hair Loss, Obesity, Stress, Thyroid disorders

ROASTED VEGETABLE AND CHICKPEA PIZZAS

Serves 6
Preparation time: 15 minutes
Cooking time: 30 minutes

1. Preheat oven to 180°C/160°C fan/gas 4.

2. In a large bowl combine the peppers, courgette and onion. Pour over the oil and add the thyme. Using your hands, mix the vegetables until well coated. Tip out onto a baking tray and roast for 15 to 20 minutes until the vegetables are tender.

3. Using the same bowl as before, add the cherry tomatoes and chickpeas and put to one side while the vegetables roast. Meanwhile, carefully using the tip of a knife pare, open each pitta bread and lay out, cut side up, on to baking sheets.

4. Remove the vegetables from the oven and add to the tomatoes and chickpeas, season with black pepper and stir well.

5. Spread the pitta breads with passata, pile the vegetable mixture on top and scatter over the cheese. Return to the oven for 8 to 10 minutes until the cheese begins to turn a pale golden colour.

6. Serve the pizzas with mixed salad leaves.

Ingredients

1 red pepper, diced
1 yellow pepper, diced
1 courgette, deseeded and sliced into sticks
1 red onion, sliced into thin wedges
1 tablepoon olive oil
1 teaspoon fresh thyme, leaves only
12 cherry tomatoes, halved
75g tinned chickpeas, rinsed and drained
6 round seeded pitta breads
175g tomato passata
100g cheddar cheese, grated
Freshly ground black pepper

To Serve

Mixed salad leaves

| Per serving: 370 kcals | 17g protein | 14g fat | 6g saturated fat | 46g carbs | 9g sugar | 8g fibre | 1.3g salt |

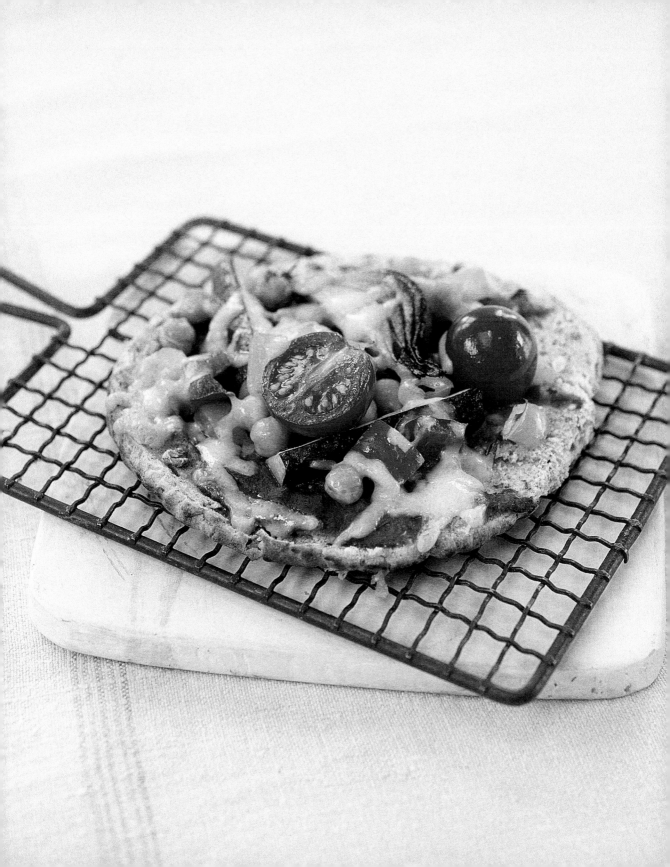

PRE-MENSTRUAL SYNDROME

PMS is an umbrella term for a host of symptoms that occur in the week (or two weeks) leading up to your period. There are over 100 symptoms commonly experienced, and most women suffer at least one, usually more, but the severity varies between women. Common ones include depression, anxiety, mood swings, irritability and tearfulness, insomnia, sugar cravings and increased appetite, fluid retention (oedema), confusion and forgetfulness, clumsiness, a swollen, bloated abdomen, breast tenderness, headaches, lower-back pain and fatigue. There is no medical test to diagnose PMS; your doctor will make the diagnosis based on the type and timing of your symptoms.

THE SCIENCE

About eight per cent of women have premenstrual symptoms that are severe enough to disrupt their lives. There are many theories about the causes of PMS, including hormonal swings in the lead-up to your period, vitamin and mineral deficiencies, low levels of the brain chemical serotonin, which affects mood and many body processes and cycles, and even very mild thyroid gland deficiency. There are many, many theories, but none has been substantiated.

Treatment can involve taking antidepressants, which raise serotonin levels; hormone treatments, such as the contraceptive pill, which regulates your cycle and can help with symptoms such as anxiety and mood swings.

Foods to Eat

- **Although not strictly a food, evening primrose oil** might help in the treatment of many symptoms of PMS. Try a daily supplement for three to four months to see if it makes a difference.

- **Other supplements to consider are vitamin B6** (found in fortified cereals, baked potatoes, bananas, chicken, pork, beef, trout and avocado; if you are taking a tablet, go for 50mg per day) and magnesium (found in spinach, pumpkin seeds, fresh soya beans, salmon, sesame seeds, white fish and pulses; supplements should contain no more than 200mg per day). These nutrients have been shown to improve a number of PMS symptoms, including those affecting your emotions.

- **Calcium-rich foods can make a difference,** and women with high levels in their diet tend to experience fewer symptoms; choose foods such as dairy produce, leafy green vegetables, soya, celery, fortified cereals, dried fruits and almonds.

Plenty of low-GL foods (including wholegrain carbohydrates), which keep blood sugar levels steady and provide a sustained source of energy, can help with cravings, irritability and mood swings, as well as sleep problems.

Fibre-rich foods, such as fresh fruit and vegetables, wholegrain carbohydrates and pulses can help to prevent constipation, and bring down oestrogen levels in your body by preventing them from being re-absorbed into your gut. It also slows down the transit of sugar in your bloodstream, which can ease the peaks and troughs that affect energy and mood.

Soya products, as well as nuts, seeds, vegetables and fruit, contain plant oestrogens, which are believed to reduce the influence of oestrogen in your body, reducing symptoms such as breast pain (see recipe on page 160).

Foods to Avoid

Sugar, salt and high levels of saturated fat are associated with bloating, breast pain and swelling.

All transfats (aka hydrogenated fats) decrease levels of prostaglandins, which work to ease inflammation and promote healthy brain function (including mood).

Caffeine causes irritability, mood swings, anxiety and irregular sleep patterns. In particular, it has been associated with breast tenderness. Avoiding caffeinated drinks in the week before your period can help to ease symptoms.

Alcohol has a negative impact on your liver, which is responsible for clearing excessive hormones (that cause hormonal imbalance) from your blood. Alcohol can also cause anxiety and depression, and swings in your blood-sugar levels.

Expert Tips

Exercising regularly can encourage the release of endorphins, which promote a feeling of wellbeing. It also works to improve your circulation, which can help with water retention and bloating.

Eat little and often; skipping meals has been shown to exacerbate PMS symptoms.

Get plenty of sleep, which can help to balance hormonal activity and reduce symptoms affecting your mood.

Try to schedule stressful events for the week after your period, when you will feel more alert and in control.

Keep a diary of your symptoms: when they begin, how severe they are, and any triggers that you can think of (i.e. was your mood worse after a couple of glasses of wine?). Not only will this help you to work out what may exacerbate or cause symptoms, but your doctor will find it useful when assessing the nature of your symptoms and deciding on the most appropriate treatment.

Smoking can make PMS symptoms worse.

WARNING

If your symptoms begin to affect your work, mood or relationships, or become unmanageable, see your doctor.

See also: Anxiety, Headaches, Insomnia, Depression.

MEDITERRANEAN SPAGHETTI

Serves 4
Preparation time: 10 minutes
Cooking time: 20 minutes

Ingredients

1. Cook the spaghetti as per pack instructions.

2. While the spaghetti is cooking, heat the oil in a large saucepan over a medium heat, add the garlic and spring onions and quickly fry for 1 to 2 minutes. Pour the tomatoes into the pan and bring up to a gentle simmer.

3. Add the capers, anchovies and soya beans to the pan and simmer for 2 minutes. Season with plenty of freshly ground black pepper. You shouldn't need any salt, as the capers and anchovies add enough salt to the dish.

4. Drain the spaghetti, reserving approximately 3 to 4 tablespoons of the pasta water to add to the sauce along with the peppers, herbs and a squeeze of lemon. Add the sauce to the spaghetti and toss well to combine. Serve immediately in warmed bowls.

400g wholewheat spaghetti
1 tablespoon olive oil
2 cloves garlic, crushed
6 spring onions, thinly sliced
400g tin cherry tomatoes
25g capers, rinsed
3 x 50g tins good-quality anchovies, drained and roughly chopped
100g frozen, podded soya beans
Freshly ground black pepper
6 pimento peppers, thinly sliced
20g bunch flat leaf parsley, leaves roughly chopped
20g bunch basil, leaves torn
Squeeze of lemon

| Per serving: 490 kcals | 29g protein | 11g fat | 1.5g saturated fat | 73g carbs | 7g sugar | 13g fibre | 5g salt |

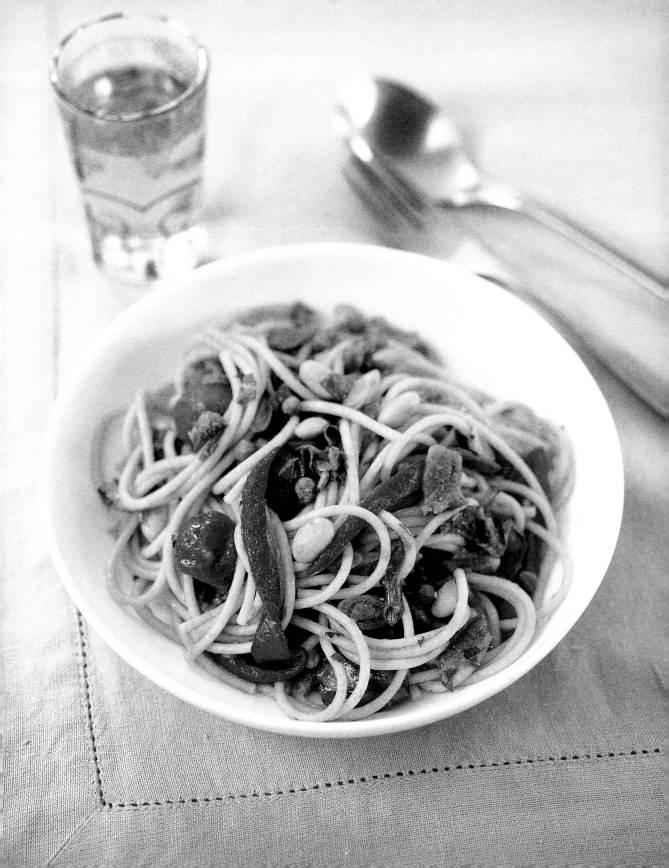

PREGNANCY

Pregnancy is a time of great excitement and emotional highs and lows, as you come to terms with the prospect of bringing a new life into the world. At no other period of your life is a healthy, balanced diet as important as it is during pregnancy. Changing your diet to include a wealth of fresh, whole foods will ensure that you get the nutrients your baby needs for optimum health and development and will protect your own health as well. What's more, you can help to avert and ease niggling – and even downright debilitating – pregnancy symptoms by making the right food choices.

Foods to Eat

- **Plenty of fresh fruit and vegetables,** which offer a host of vitamins and minerals, as well as fibre, which encourages optimum absorption of nutrients from the foods you eat, and helps to prevent constipation.

- **Good-quality animal and plant proteins** (such as lean meats, poultry, dairy products, fish, eggs, nuts, seeds, lentils and other pulses, and soya), which are necessary for the development of every new cell in your baby's body.

- **Whole, unrefined carbohydrates** (such as wholegrain pasta and bread, wild or brown rice, potatoes and pulses) to keep your blood sugar levels steady, provide you with energy and fibre, and supply key nutrients for your baby's development.

- **Lean red meats, leafy green vegetables, fish, dried fruit, beets, molasses, wholegrain bread, and iron-fortified cereals,** which offer plenty of iron to prevent anaemia in you (common during pregnancy), and ensure that your baby develops adequate stores.

- **Dairy produce, soya, almonds and leafy green vegetables,** which are a good source of calcium, required for your baby's bones and teeth – and yours.

- **Nuts, seeds, oily fish (such as salmon and mackerel; but see below), avocados and eggs.** These contain essential fatty acids (EFAs) necessary for the development of your baby's brain and nervous system.

- **Dark green vegetables, nuts, Marmite, brown rice, fortified breakfast cereals and whole grains,** which contain folic acid that can help to prevent neural tube defects, such as spina bifida (see page 164).

Foods to Avoid

- **Liver and cod liver oil** (which can provide too much of the animal form of vitamin A, which is linked to birth defects).

- **Too much oily fish,** which can contain pollutants such as dioxins, mercury and PCBs; stick to two servings of fresh oily fish and no more than four cans of tuna a week. Avoid shark, swordfish and marlin altogether.

- **Raw seafood,** which can contain parasites and bacteria; sushi that has been made with smoked or previously frozen fish or shellfish is fine.

- **Unpasteurized soft or blue cheese,** such as camembert, goat's cheese, brie and stilton (these can contain listeria).

- **Raw or partially cooked eggs,** including homemade mayonnaise (which can contain salmonella).

- **Raw or undercooked meat, fish and poultry** (these can contain salmonella or *Toxoplasma gondii*, which causes toxoplasmosis).

- **Ready-to-eat-salads in bags** (because of the risk of listeria).

- **Meat pâtés** (which can bring on food-borne illnesses).

- **Alcohol,** which can cross the placenta and affect your baby's development. It's best to avoid it altogether but if you choose to drink have no more than one or two glasses a week.

- **More than 200mg of caffeine** (about two cups of strong tea or instant coffee, or 1.5 cups of filter coffee) per day; excess caffeine is linked with miscarriage and low birth weight.

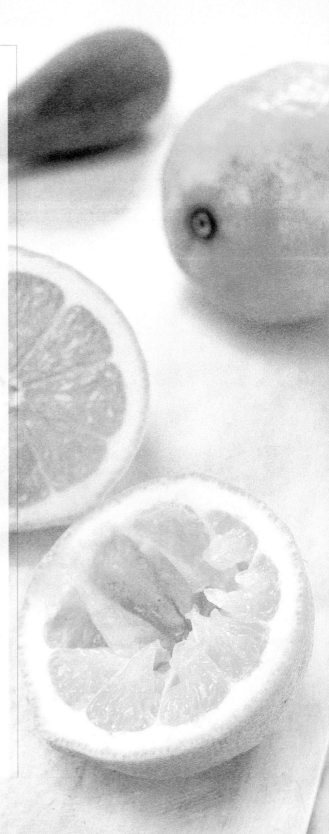

DO I NEED SUPPLEMENTS?

You'll need 400mcg of folic acid per day, taken in tablet form, every day while you are trying to conceive and until you are twelve weeks pregnant. Some women will need higher levels; for example, if you have diabetes, take medication for epilepsy or suffer from coeliac disease. This helps to prevent neural tube defects, heart defects, cleft lip and palate and a premature birth.

EATING FOR TWO

Gone are the days when mums were encouraged to eat twice as much as they did before pregnancy. In fact, we now know that pregnant women do not need to increase their calorie intake until the third trimester, when only 200 additional calories may be required each day to sustain your baby's growth – and your energy levels – and help to maintain a healthy weight. Two hundred calories amounts to a small sandwich or a couple of pieces of fruit and a small chunk of cheese. If you are carrying twins, you will need about 600 more calories per day. Putting on weight is a necessary part of pregnancy, and you can expect to gain an average of 12.5kg (27.6lbs), although this varies a great deal between women.

PREGNANCY SYMPTOMS

There is plenty of research to suggest that a healthy diet can help to prevent unpleasant symptoms, or at least reduce their severity. What's more, a balanced diet can make you feel more relaxed and in control.

MORNING SICKNESS:

Pregnancy-related nausea and vomiting can occur at any time of the day, so it is important to maximize your food intake when you feel well enough to eat. Staying hydrated is also important, to reduce symptoms and protect your health and that of your baby.

- **Dry biscuits seem to help ease nausea:** go for nutritious wholegrain biscuits (with seeds, if possible) for maximum nutrition.

- **Ginger is a traditional remedy for morning sickness:** you can drink ginger tea (see recipe on page 165), chew crystallized or candied ginger, or nibble ginger biscuits until symptoms pass.

- **Peppermint tea may help** to settle your tummy, as it improves digestion.

Oedema (water retention):

The additional fluid retained during pregnancy can collect around your feet, ankles, and even your fingers and face.

- **Asparagus, lemons, parsley, melon, beets, cucumber, watercress and artichokes are all natural diuretics,** which promote urination and encourage the function of your kidneys.

- **Fresh herbal teas** (such as fennel and dandelion) will help to flush out excess water; drinking plenty of fresh water will also help to reduce water retention.

- **Flavour foods** with herbs and spices, rather than salt, which can cause oedema.

Mood swings:

Although hormonal changes are at the root of mood swings, tearfulness, irritability and anxiety, including particular foods in your diet can help to ease them.

- **Eat plenty of wholegrain carbohydrates,** which stabilize your blood sugar and help to prevent surges and dips that can affect your mood. Oats are particularly good, as they provide sustained energy and also contain B vitamins, which can encourage the health of your nervous system.

Expert Tips

- **A good breakfast will give you the ideal start to the day,** while a small snack before bed can encourage restful sleep and help to prevent nausea upon rising the next morning.

- **Eating little and often can ease nausea,** provide energy and reduce cravings.

- **Always eat a piece of fruit or drink a little orange** (or other fruit) juice with meals, to ensure that any iron contained in your food is better absorbed.

- **Regular exercise can help to keep your weight stable,** encourage circulation, ease muscular aches and pains and oedema, and also help to reduce your risk of obesity-related pregnancy problems, such as pre-eclampsia.

CASE STUDY

*M*andy suffered from heartburn in the second and third trimesters of her pregnancy, as her growing baby put pressure on her stomach, causing the acid to rise into her oesophagus. She reduced fatty foods in her diet, cut out caffeine and fizzy drinks, and ate several small meals each day, which had a big impact upon her symptoms. Best of all, she found that eating a little fresh pineapple or papaya (which encourage digestion and reduces stomach acid) before meals alleviated the problem.

WARNING

See your doctor if you experience any unusual symptoms. In particular, bleeding, cramping, headaches, vision changes or extreme vomiting should be reported immediately.

See also: Constipation, Fatigue, Haemorrhoids, Headaches, Indigestion/Heartburn, Insomnia

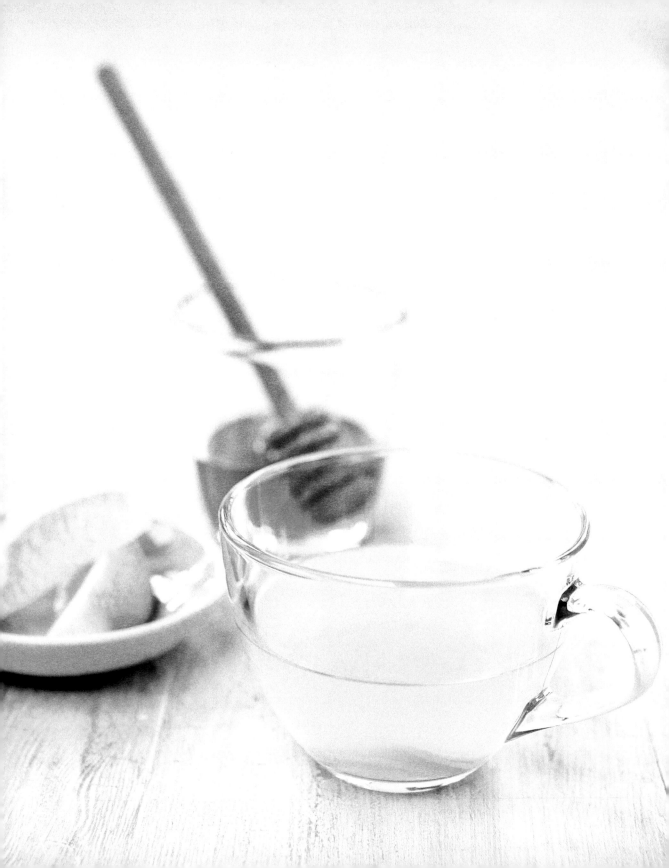

GINGER TEA WITH HONEY AND LEMON

Makes 2 mugs

Ingredients

1. Place the ginger in a small saucepan and pour over 500ml water, bring to a simmer for 5 minutes. Add the lemon and honey, if liked, stir and taste.

   The ginger water can be made in advance and drunk hot or chilled, whichever helps.

5cm piece of fresh root ginger, peeled and sliced
Juice of ½ lemon, optional
1–2 teaspoons runny honey, optional

Per serving: 17 kcals | 0g protein | 0g fat | 0g saturated fat | 4g carbs | 4g sugar | 0g fibre | 0g salt

VAGINAL ODOUR

Vaginal odour is a symptom of other health conditions, rather than a health problem in its own right, but it can be extremely embarrassing for sufferers. It's worth noting that the vagina is self-cleaning, so odour is not usually a sign of poor hygiene. It is normally caused by thrush, bacterial vaginosis (a bacterial imbalance in the vagina), or trichomoniasis (a sexually transmitted illness (STI) caused by a parasite). There are other potential causes, such as pelvic inflammatory disease (PID), and several STIs. Your doctor will diagnose the cause by taking a swab of your vagina, and sending it to a laboratory for testing.

THE SCIENCE

There are a number of different conditions that can lead to vaginal odour, each of which has its own causes. Treatment will be based on the cause, so antibiotics may be suggested for infections and some STIs, while anti-thrush medication may be useful for thrush. In some cases, a weakened immune system, poor diet and an imbalance in the pH balance of your vagina may be at the root.

Foods to Eat

- **Probiotic drinks and yoghurts** will help to promote the health of good bacteria in your body, which will prevent bad bacteria from developing. What's more, foods containing lactobacillus help to establish a healthier pH balance in your vagina, which can reduce odour.
- **Stick to a low-GL diet whenever possible,** as insulin resistance (see Diabetes, page 232) may be linked with vaginal odour.
- **Foods high in beta-carotene** will help to prevent the spread of infection, and encourage the health of your vagina.
- **Garlic** has strong anti-bacterial properties; eating it raw or lightly roasted can keep infection at bay.

Foods to Avoid

- **Alcohol can feed any bacteria at the root of the problem,** which change the pH balance of your vagina, making it more susceptible to infection, and lower your immunity.
- **Sugar in excess** can cause bacteria to breed, causing odour.

Expert Tips

- **Avoid perfumes, sprays and harsh washing products,** which can upset the pH balance of your vagina, as well as the balance of healthy bacteria.
- **Avoid tight trousers or underwear** as these can rub and cause inflammation.
- **Use condoms when you have sex**, which reduces the likelihood of acquiring an STI, and also protects your body from contact with sperm, which can upset the pH balance of your vagina.

WARNING

Report any sign of infection (including foul-smelling or unusual discharge) to your doctor, particularly if it is accompanied by fever.

See also: Vaginal thrush

VAGINAL THRUSH

Seventy-five per cent of women will experience thrush at some point in their lives. This fungal infection causes irritation and swelling of the vagina and vulva, and is commonly known as a 'yeast infection' or 'candida'. Symptoms can include itching, a sore vulva, pain during intercourse and/or urination and a vaginal discharge (thin and watery, or thick and white). A diagnosis is usually made on the basis of your symptoms, but sometimes tests are required. These can include taking a swab of your vaginal secretions, which is then assessed in a laboratory, and having the pH balance of your vagina tested.

THE SCIENCE

Thrush is mainly caused by high levels of candida in the body, which can be caused by a poor diet (particularly one that is high in sugar and refined carbohydrates), stress and oral contraceptives. Antibiotics affect the normal bacterial flora in the vagina, predisposing to thrush. Treatment can include an anti-thrush pessary (placed in your vagina), creams, or tablets that are taken orally.

Foods to Eat

- **Eat plenty of orange and yellow fruits and vegetables,** which contain beta-carotene. This helps to support the health of your vagina (by improving mucous membranes), and can help to prevent and treat yeast infections.
- **Apple cider vinegar** (unlike all other vinegars) can help to combat a yeast infection when diluted and used on your vagina to soothe and balance.

Foods to Avoid

- **Sugar of all descriptions** (including that found in alcohol) will feed candida, and cause it to flourish.
- **Avoid yeasty foods** including bread, Marmite, beer and vinegar, which can cause inflammation of your gut and encourage overgrowth.
- **Fermented foods,** such as vinegar.

Expert Tips

- **Avoid douching and using perfumes** or other products in the vaginal area, which can upset the pH balance of your vagina.
- **Wear cotton underwear,** which allows the area to breathe and discourages the build-up of fungi.
- **Change tampons regularly,** to avoid the area becoming too warm and moist.
- **Take steps to reduce stress** by exercising regularly and getting plenty of sleep and relaxation; stress has been linked with thrush.
- **Avoid using latex condoms,** spermicidal creams or lubricants, which can irritate your vagina.

WARNING

If you suffer from pain, itching or a foul-smelling discharge, see your doctor.

See also: Vaginal odour

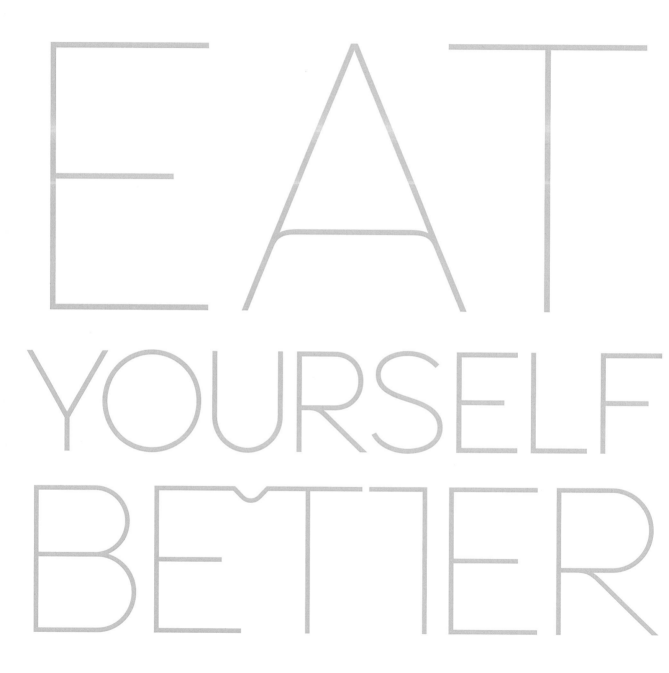

Fifty years ago we went straight to the doctor if anything was wrong with us and were prescribed some tablets – antibiotics, maybe, or antihistamines. We didn't ask questions but took them as instructed, then sat back and waited for them to work. It's almost as though we'd handed over control of our health. In the last couple of decades, though, television programmes, books and Sunday supplement articles have given us enough information to take back a measure of that control. We still need to go to the doctor if we have any troubling symptoms, but we can take steps to heal ourselves as well.

The food we eat is a major factor in determining how we feel now, and how we will feel in the future. Of course, other lifestyle issues are important, such as taking more exercise, but these changes are much easier to implement when we know what we are doing and why we are doing it, rather than simply being told to move about more. And the same applies to what we eat and drink.

In the past, there was a small minority who recognized that nutrition played an important part in their health, and that they could address what was wrong through what they ate, but they were often dismissed as the 'knit-your-own-yoghurt' brigade: cranks inclined to gritty brown rice and stodgy vegetarian dishes. That's no longer the case; the importance of nutrition in the causes and treatment of various complaints has passed into the scientific mainstream, and reliable new research is appearing almost every day. Food really can play a key part in the prevention, amelioration and treatment of a whole range of comparatively minor problems.

If we need any further incentive to take back some of the control over our own health, we can bear in mind that a varied healthy diet – one with a wide range of essential nutrients – can make all of us feel fundamentally better. And healthy food tastes delicious, too; the days of the four-ton veggie burger have gone. Now there's an added incentive!

BURNS

We automatically think of fires as being the main cause of burns, but of course there are others: the sun, some chemicals (including hair products), hot liquids, ice-cold metal, friction (think rope burns) and electrical contact. There are different degrees – literally – of burns, depending on how deep they go, and the pain you experience may not reflect the seriousness of the burn. Deep burns destroy the nerves, making the area numb, while shallower ones damage them – and that's why small burns can be so excruciating.

THE SCIENCE

The skin is your body's biggest organ, and it has three layers. The epidermis is the outermost one; then comes the dermis, which has hair follicles, sweat glands, tiny blood vessels and nerves. The final layer is the subcutaneous fat which contains nerves and bigger blood vessels, and keeps you from overheating or getting too cold.

First-degree burns affecting the epidermis only are often called superficial burns, but that refers to the depth of the burn, not the seriousness. If you've been sunburnt, this is probably the type of burn you've experienced. Your skin will be red and painful and you may have some swelling where you've been burnt, but no blistering. Treat the burnt areas with cold packs and maybe aloe vera gel, and they won't scar. If children are the ones with the burns, see a medic, as they can get sick more quickly with sunburn than adults.

Second-degree or partial-thickness burns involve the epidermis and the dermis. These are also generally painful – the nerves are still intact – but blisters are likely to appear. No matter how tempting it may be, do not pop these; you need medical help. These burns can result in scars. Third-degree burns – full-thickness burns – are the most severe. There's a loss of sensation and

a very high chance of infection, so get emergency medical attention immediately.

There are some basic rules for second-degree burns: don't touch the burn, and don't pull off or peel any loose skin or burst blisters. Cooling the area that has been burned is a priority, so hold the burnt part of the body under cold running water for ten minutes. Avoid creams and ointments unless prescribed by your doctor. Don't use plasters or soft dressings; use a dampened sterile dressing, a plastic bag or clean cling film to wrap over the burn instead, and then get medical help. For a liquid burn, immediately remove any clothing where the liquid was spilled or the area might continue to burn, then immerse the burn in cold water.

The next stage is recovery. For all levels of burn, make sure you drink plenty of water and keep hydrated. It takes a lot of energy for the body to repair itself, so people with more serious burns need extra calories to aid wound recovery. A healthy, varied diet should provide all the iron, zinc, vitamin C and antioxidants you need, plus plenty of protein to heal subcutaneous tissues and repair damaged collagen.

Foods to Eat

- **Lots of water** for hydration.
- **Protein** to help deep healing: lean meat, fish, dairy products such as yoghurt and milk, eggs (they'll also help boost zinc and potassium levels).
- **Fresh fruit and green leafy vegetables** for their vitamin and antioxidant content.

Foods to Avoid

- **Caffeine** – that's tea, coffee, and many fizzy drinks: caffeine is a diuretic, and you need to boost hydration levels, not deplete them.
- **Alcohol,** because the same applies.

Expert Tip

- **Don't forget to drink lots of water** and keep hydrated if you're in the sun; dehydration is one of the fundamental reasons why people get sunstroke.

WARNING

Burns can be fatal and sometimes hidden if they affect the airway. What we've written here is basic first aid. You should always see a doctor if a child has burns.

With any burns, if there are symptoms of shock, such as rapid heartbeat, dizziness, mental confusion or loss of consciousness, don't hesitate to get emergency help.

Burns from sunbathing can be serious. And not only does sunbathing speed up skin ageing, but it is also directly linked to developing skin cancer, and that's a killer. Always use high-factor sunscreen and be sensible about exposure. You can get sunburn on a sunbed just as easily as on a beach, and they're best avoided, because the UV rays are delivered in a way that is particularly dangerous.

See also: Cancer, Wrinkles/ageing skin

COLDS AND COUGHS

Winter is the prime time for colds and coughs, but no research has definitively explained exactly why this is. More than ninety per cent are caused by viruses – there are over 200 that can cause colds – and won't respond to antibiotics. There are different types of coughs – dry and chesty. Inflammation causes dry coughs, and with chesty coughs there is phlegm.

There are several things you can do to help yourself when you're suffering, and some that may reduce the likelihood of you succumbing to any colds and coughs that are doing the rounds in the first place. But it's worth remembering, especially when you're feeling terrible, that coughs and colds usually get better by themselves without the need for any treatment.

THE SCIENCE

Colds and coughs are very contagious. On average, adults have between two and four colds a year, children between six and eight. Women get more than men (probably because they're often in closer contact with children). They can be spread either directly, by small droplets released when you sneeze or cough, or indirectly: if you were to cough on to your hand and use a handrail, for instance, and someone used the rail after you and then touched their own mouth or nose, they could catch your cold. When your symptoms are bad, you're very contagious, but you are also contagious just before the symptoms show.

Many people take vitamin C supplements to prevent colds and coughs, but it's controversial and has been for years. There's not a lot of solid scientific evidence supporting it; in fact, it's rather the opposite – studies involving 11,300 people found that taking vitamin C tablets failed to reduce the incidence of colds. It's far better to get vitamin C from food. When you're doing that, you're getting a range of valuable antioxidants, not just vitamin C, and vitamins from foods are likely to be easier for the body to access (they are more 'bio-available').

Some people swear by the herbal remedy echinacea for preventing and treating colds. There have been some research studies but the evidence is inconclusive to date. Garlic is interesting, because a study of 146 people showed that those who ate some garlic every day for three months caught fewer colds. If they caught a cold it didn't reduce the effects, but they weren't as likely to catch colds in the first place. Garlic has antimicrobial and antiviral properties, so that might be why it works.

Several studies indicate that zinc is a significant factor in both preventing and alleviating colds, but there can be side effects if you take zinc supplements long term. It's far better to make sure you are eating lots of zinc-containing foods as the cold season approaches.

Foods to Eat

- **Stay well hydrated.** Hot drinks are especially good as the steam can help to loosen mucus.
- **Boost your vitamin C** with lots of lovely vegetables and fruit, and not just oranges. Pineapple, mango, kiwi fruit, berries and guava are all high in vitamin C.
- **Seafood** is a good source of zinc, as are dairy products, Brazil nuts, eggs and poultry.
- **Garlic,** because of its antiviral properties, may help reduce the number of colds you get. Make your own wholegrain garlic bread, add garlic to soups, casseroles and stir-fries, or have lots in a pasta sauce.

Foods to Avoid

- **Milk** seems to increase mucus production in some people and it can also make the phlegm thicker and more irritating. But if you are using a milk substitute such as soya milk, make sure it is fortified with calcium so you are not missing out.

Expert Tips

- **Soup is a good choice** when you've got a cold and may have lost your appetite. Nutrients from meat, vegetables and pulses are retained in the liquid and it's easy to make a decent soup at home even if you are not an experienced cook. Chicken soup has anti-inflammatory properties, which helps ease upper respiratory infections (see recipe on page 176).
- **It can be tempting to buy every cold remedy going** when you're feeling miserable, and there's no harm in using them sparingly, but be very careful if mixing them that you don't inadvertently take an overdose of paracetamol, which is in many over-the-counter medications.

WARNING

There are several reasons to see your doctor with a bad cold: if you're elderly or if it's a young child who's sneezing and coughing; if the fever doesn't go even though you've taken paracetamol; if you're coughing up thick mucus which is green, yellow or blood-stained; if you're wheezing or short of breath; if you've been abroad; or if you've got another health condition (such as diabetes, asthma or kidney disease).

See your doctor if a cough doesn't clear up, or if it gets worse over about a fortnight even though your other symptoms have improved.

See also: Asthma, Hay fever, Influenza, Sinusitis

CHICKEN AND MIXED VEGETABLE SOUP

Serves 4
Preparation time: 10 minutes
Cooking time: 2½ hours

1. Tip all of the ingredients into a very large pan or stock pot, cover with cold water and bring to a gentle simmer. Simmer uncovered for 2½ hours; every 30 minutes or so you should skim off any fat or scum from the surface.

2. Carefully remove and discard the chicken carcass, wings, thyme stems and bay leaves from the soup. Using a hand-held stick blender, carefully blend the soup until smooth. Season to taste with a touch of salt and plenty of freshly ground black pepper. Serve with thick, crusty wholemeal bread.

Ingredients

1 raw chicken carcass – from the butcher
1kg chicken wings
1 onion, peeled and quartered
1 leek, sliced into chunks
1 sweet potato, peeled and quartered
2 parsnips, scrubbed and halved
2 turnips, scrubbed and halved
½ celeriac, peeled and cut into 5cm cubes
6 carrots, peeled and halved
2 sticks celery
1 x 20g bunch flat leaf parsley
8 stems thyme
2 bay leaves

| Per serving: 210 kcals | 4g protein | 7g fat | 1g saturated fat | 34g carbs | 20g sugar | 14g fibre | 0.3g salt |

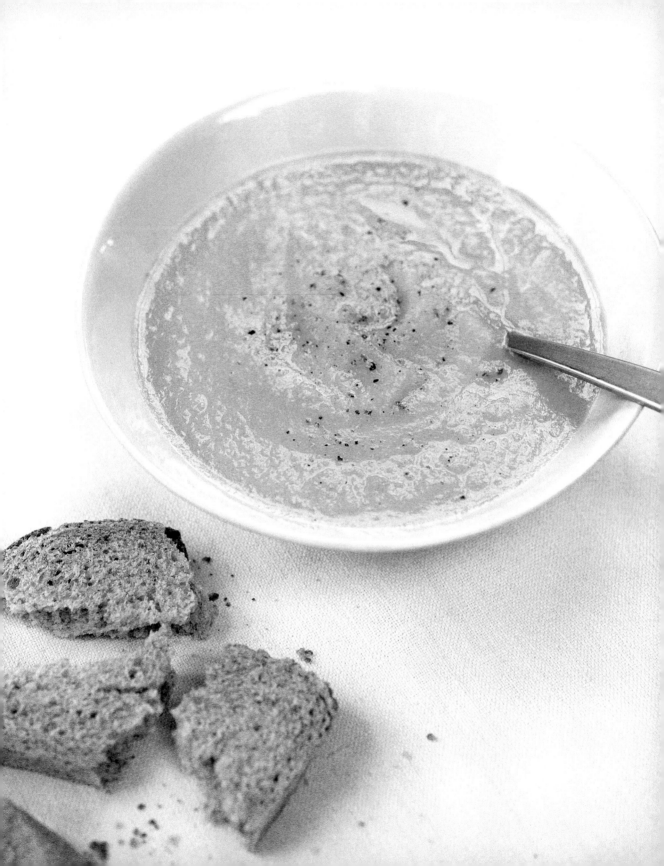

CYSTITIS

During an attack of cystitis you want to urinate frequently and feel you need to do so urgently, but when you get to the toilet you may not produce much liquid. Urination can cause stinging pain, and there can sometimes be blood in the urine (which is alarming but probably not serious). You might also experience lower abdominal pain and a high temperature. Most cystitis either clears up on its own, once you know what to do for yourself, or it may need a course of antibiotics.

THE SCIENCE

When you have cystitis, your bladder is inflamed. This is usually because of an infection, but irritation and damage can also play a part. It's generally caused by the bacteria which live quite harmlessly on the skin, finding their way up along the urethra and into the bladder (the urethra is very close to the anus, which doesn't help). Woman get cystitis more than men because their urethras are shorter, and changes in oestrogen levels affecting the tissues after the menopause make older women more vulnerable. Urinary-tract infections (UTIs) such as cystitis are more common if you're pregnant, too, because

of hormonal changes – and if this is the case you should get medical advice because there's an increased risk of miscarriage. Some women are especially prone to cystitis because they have a shorter urethra than most, and bacteria can reach the bladder more easily.

The blood that some sufferers see when they urinate is because the bladder is so inflamed that it actually bleeds. If you've got blood in your urine and no other UTI symptoms, see your GP straight away, and go again if it persists after your cystitis has cleared up. Go to your doctor if you get recurring cystitis as well, because it can be linked to kidney stones and other urinary tract problems. Cystitis is hard to treat effectively without antibiotics once it has really taken hold, but there are things you can do to mitigate the effects or help prevent attacks in the first place.

The most useful thing you can do when you're in the middle of a cystitis attack is to drink loads and loads of plain water. Cranberries can help to prevent attacks, because substances they contain seem to play a role in preventing the bacteria from sticking to the bladder wall, so they are worth including in your diet if you are susceptible.

It's important to try to prevent bacteria entering the urethra, so wipe yourself front to back when you've been to the toilet and avoid using sprays or powders. Don't use perfumed soaps, bubble baths and body washes either, as chemical irritants can be a factor in getting cystitis. Create an unfriendly atmosphere for bacteria: shower rather than bathe, wear cotton underwear, and don't hold out if you need to urinate, as doing so can put extra stress on the bladder. Sex (oral as well as genital) may play a role in introducing bacteria into the urethra, and it can also cause irritation. Wash before having sex, use a lubricant if you need to, and wash afterwards – hands as well!

- **As soon as you notice the first signs of cystitis,** start drinking lots and lots of water.

- **For prevention,** you can take cranberry capsules if you don't like the taste of the juice. Cranberries have a sharp taste and are often over-sweetened in shop-bought juices to compensate. Check the ingredients information on juice packaging if you react to artificial sweeteners. Alternatively, make your own cranberry juice following our recipe (see page 180).

- **Alcohol and drinks containing a lot of caffeine (tea, coffee, cola) will make you dehydrated,** so cut them out during an attack and only drink them in moderation the rest of the time.

- **Some people have reported that spicy food can trigger an attack.** If you get recurrent cystitis, keeping a food and symptom diary may help you work out if there are triggers involved.

- **If you are prone to getting cystitis,** try to avoid having sex after drinking a lot of alcohol. Yes, we know this might be difficult for some, but the combination of the dehydrating effect of the booze plus friction is a sure-fire recipe for a cystitis infection.

- **Empty your bladder before and after sex** as stagnant urine is the perfect breeding ground for bacteria.

WARNING

A child with a urine infection needs to see a doctor urgently for further investigation. Men should also see their GP, as should women having their first attack. And if you have symptoms that last more than three days, don't tough it out; go and get a prescription for antibiotics, as the infection can spread to the kidneys or cause sepsis.

Unexplained blood in your urine – especially without any other symptoms – should always be checked out by your GP.

See also: Kidney stones, Pregnancy, Menopause

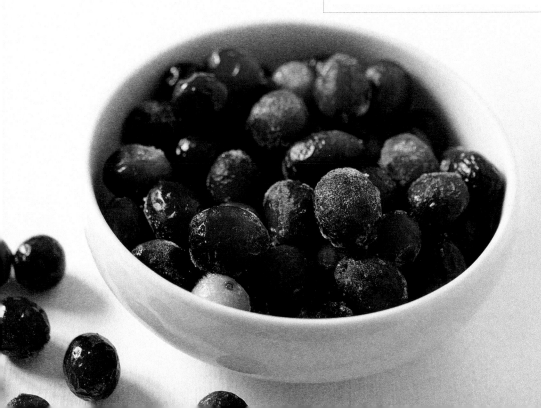

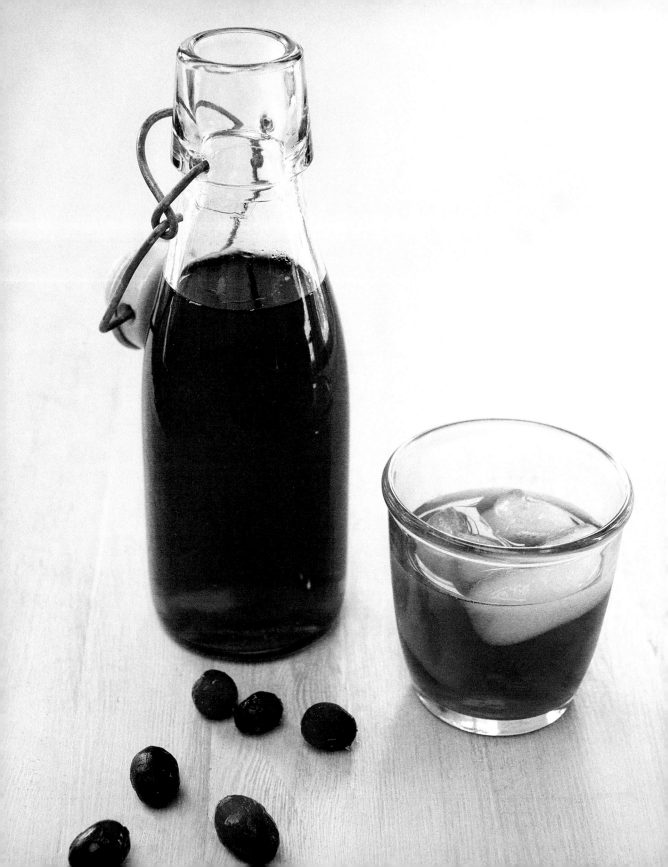

HOMEMADE CRANBERRY JUICE

Makes 1 litre (150ml serving)
Cooking time: 20 minutes

Ingredients

1. Tip the cranberries and 1.2 litres water into a large non-reactive pan, bring to a gentle simmer and cook for 15 minutes or until the berries start to burst.

2. Strain the cranberries through a colander placed over another large non-reactive pan.

3. Add sugar to taste and return to a gentle heat until the sugar dissolves.

4. Carefully pour into clean glass bottles and leave to cool before refrigerating.

500g frozen cranberries
75g unrefined caster sugar

| 150ml serving: 37 kcals | 0g protein | 0g fat | 0g saturated fat | 10g carbs | 10g sugar | 0g fibre | trace salt |

ERECTILE DYSFUNCTION

Suffering with erectile dysfunction can be miserable, isolating and depressing, for both you and your partner. But you are far from being alone – about half of all men between the ages of forty and seventy will have some degree of ED. It's quite normal and may simply be because older men require more stimulation than an eighteen-year-old does. Sometimes ED can be subjective, and this is particularly true of younger men who may have unrealistic expectations (thanks, pornography!). So don't feel embarrassed and alone; get help and support instead.

THE SCIENCE

When you become aroused, the nerves in your penis increase the blood flow, which makes the tissue expand and harden. Erectile dysfunction is simply defined as the inability to get enough of an erection to have sex. This covers every degree from nothing at all happening to having unsustained erections or erections which you don't think are firm enough. Because of the basic mechanics, erection problems can be caused by anything that interferes with your circulation (blocked arteries mean reduced blood flow, and that means not much of an erection) or nervous system (the nerves don't fire properly, so don't initiate the changes necessary to increase blood flow to the penis). Sometimes it's directly related to 'performance anxiety' because you're in a new relationship, or have unrealistic expectations. ED can also be associated with having a low level of sexual desire – a low libido. Some medication can also cause ED, as can alcohol and certain street drugs.

With such a diverse set of possibilities, it's clear that there's no single solution that will suit everyone, but that should be encouraging – there are a lot of potential solutions to explore, and no reason to give up before you even seek help. But because there are so many possible explanations, and because there may be other things going on which can have serious implications (such as more general problems with your blood vessels), it is important to get that help.

Smokers and heavy drinkers are more likely to suffer from ED than others. Obesity is also a factor. There's some encouraging news here: change your diet to one which includes Mediterranean elements and you may well see a significant improvement over time, because it will improve circulation, lower cholesterol, and you should also lose some weight.

Exercise can help, as can your GP: there are drugs that he or she can prescribe, such as PDE-5 inhibitors (Pfizer's Viagra is probably the best known), but you should be monitored while taking them and they may not be suitable if you have underlying health problems. Don't buy them over the internet without seeing your doctor, because apart from anything else, you will have no idea what you're actually getting – and taking nitrates for heart disease at the same time as drugs like Viagra can be fatal.

Foods to Eat

- **The Mediterranean diet is recommended** because it can have a powerful impact on your circulation and overall health. That means eating lots of fresh fruit and vegetables, whole grains (so wholemeal bread, etc.), lots of fish and seafood (particularly good for zinc) and, classically, olive oil and tomatoes.
- **In a small study, eating 100g of pistachio nuts a day over three weeks improved participants' ED (and the level of healthy fats in their blood).** That's quite a lot of nuts, and quite a lot of calories, so you'd have to replace some of your food or you'd put on too much weight – but it's a thought (see recipe on page 184).
- **Watermelon –** some say this is the Viagra of fruits.

Foods to Avoid

- **Booze.** Keep alcohol intake low (most men are all too aware of the consequences of too much drink, but you can forget after a couple of pints), and go for small amounts of red wine instead of large amounts of beer.
- **Keep red meat to a minimum** – that's part of the Mediterranean diet.
- **Cut back on salt:** vital if you've got high blood pressure.

Expert Tip

- **Be very, very careful about the medications and bizarre treatments often found online.** This is an area that attracts 'snake-oil salesmen' (and plenty of fake look-a-like products), so talk to your GP first.

WARNING

It's important to see your doctor to rule out or deal with any serious issues which might underlie your ED, whether that's something like diabetes or depression, a drug you've been prescribed, or a neurological disorder.

Taking erectile drugs (like Viagra) with prescribed nitrates can be fatal.

See also: Cardiovascular disease, Diabetes, High blood pressure, High cholesterol, Infertility, Sex drive – lack of

CHILLI PORK CHOPS WITH STIR-FRIED VEGETABLES AND COUSCOUS

Serves 4
Preparation time: 20 minutes
Cooking time: 15 minutes

1. Preheat grill to a high heat.

2. Mix half the oil, half the lemon and the paprika and chilli powder together in a small bowl, brush on to the pork chops and grill for 7 minutes each side or until cooked through.

3. Meanwhile, pour the couscous into a large bowl and pour over the hot stock, cover the bowl with clingfilm and set aside for 5 minutes.

4. Heat the remaining olive oil in a large pan or wok and quickly stir-fry the mangetout or sugarsnap peas for 1 minute, add the peas and stir-fry for a further 2 minutes.

5. Fluff up the couscous with a fork and stir through the remaining lemon, the herbs, pistachio nuts, tomatoes and peppers. Season to taste with freshly ground black pepper and serve with the pork chops.

Ingredients

1 tablespoon olive oil

Juice and grated zest of 1 lemon

1½ teaspoons paprika

1 teaspoon medium chilli powder

4 pork chops, with all visible fat removed

300g couscous

350ml hot chicken or vegetable reduced-sodium stock

200g mangetout or sugarsnap peas

150g frozen petits pois

20g flat leaf parsley, leaves only and roughly chopped

20g basil, leaves only and roughly torn

100g pistachio nuts, roughly chopped

8 cherry tomatoes, halved

100g roasted peppers in olive oil, drained and sliced

Freshly ground black pepper

Per serving: 591 kcals | 48g protein | 23g fat | 4g saturated fat | 53g carbs | 6g sugar | 6g fibre | 0.3g salt

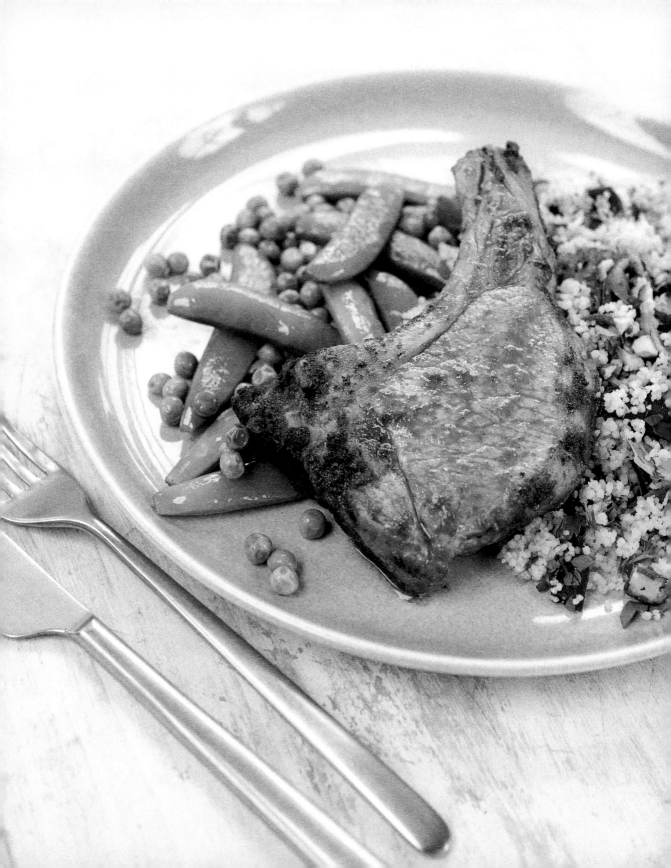

EYESIGHT, DETERIORATION OF

It's sad but true: our eyesight deteriorates with age, so it's perfectly normal to need reading glasses by your fifties. Visit an optician as soon as you notice that you're having difficulty reading the small print on labels; you can buy reading glasses over the counter, but it's worth getting a specific diagnosis initially. Other causes of deteriorating eyesight include age-related macular degeneration or AMD, cataracts and glaucoma. If you are diabetic, controlling your blood sugar levels will reduce your risk of cataracts.

THE SCIENCE

If you're developing AMD, then you will begin to notice that you're finding it difficult to see what's directly in front of you. That's because the macula, which is responsible for central vision, isn't functioning as it was, and you need central vision for reading, driving and watching TV. There are two kinds of AMD: wet and dry. If you have either of these you should be under the care of a specialist and usually require long-term follow-up. AMD is associated with smoking (and the risk is still there, even fifteen years after you've given up) and having a high BMI. There's also some evidence of a link with a high intake of saturated fats, which probably accounts for the BMI factor – the more saturated fats in your diet, the higher your BMI is likely to be.

Cataracts are cloudy patches within the transparent lens in front of the eye. As the cataracts grow, less and less light gets to the back of the eye. The cloudier the lens, the worse the effect on your sight. They need to be treated; though brighter light and strong glasses or magnifiers can help, untreated cataracts can result in blindness. If cataracts are interfering with your everyday life, your GP is likely to recommend surgery. Cataract removal is a common procedure and is usually very successful, so don't worry about it!

Glaucoma is increased pressure in the eyeball. Your optitican will be able to spot any pressure changes in the eye before you experience any symptoms.

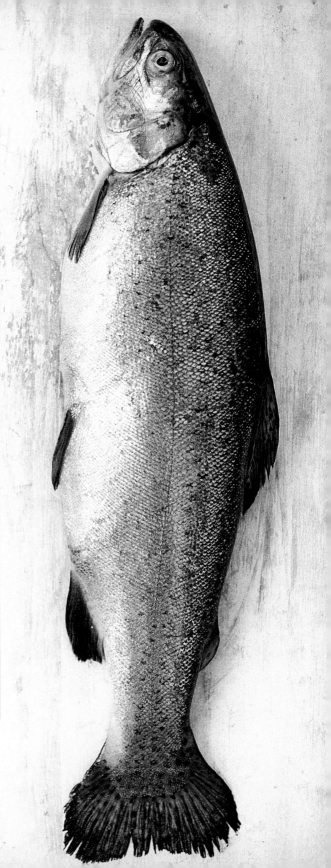

Foods to Eat

- **Those who eat a lot of fish have a twelve per cent lower risk of developing cataracts,** and it seems to help reduce AMD risk too.

- **Make sure you eat lots of fresh fruit and vegetables,** especially greens. Carotenoids and lutein are really important for the health of your eyes, and they're found in things like spinach and kale. Blueberries are also excellent sources.

Foods to Avoid

- **Reduce your fat intake overall and steer clear of saturated fat as far as possible.** That means no processed biscuits and cakes, as they're especially high. Cut back on red meat and full-fat dairy products. Always take the skin off poultry and trim the fat off other meat before cooking, to reduce the amount of saturated fat.

- **Don't take a supplement of vitamins A or C if you're a smoker.** It's always best to get the nutrients your body needs through your diet anyway, but carotenoid supplements can actually *increase* the risk of smokers developing lung cancer.

Expert Tips

- **Focus on getting lots of monounsaturated fats,** especially omega 3.
- **Take fish oil supplements** if you really can't stand fish.
- **Some polyunsaturates can also help** to protect you from AMD.

WARNING

Any visual disturbances need to be checked out by your doctor.

See also: High cholesterol, Smoking

GOUT

Gout may sound rather Victorian, but it's actually the most common type of inflammatory arthritis. It's particularly common in people who are overweight and especially men. Symptoms include joint inflammation and swelling. If you've a red, painful, swollen big toe, it could be gout because that's the most common part of the body affected (although it can strike ankles, knees, wrists, fingers and elbows). The pain can be sudden and agonizing, but it can be treated with a combination of medicine and lifestyle changes.

THE SCIENCE

There's a hereditary element, but it's not a very clear one. What *is* clear is that gout is caused by uric acid building up in the body. It's normally excreted by the kidneys, but when too much is produced or too little removed, crystals can accumulate in the joints and cause inflammation. It's connected to the body breaking down purines, chemicals found in alcohol and some foods such as meat and fish (purines are found in other foods, but it's those from meat and fish that seem to affect gout the most).

Treating gout involves dealing with the symptoms of an attack, and trying to reduce the likelihood of further attacks. Some things you can do yourself – using ice packs to relieve the inflammation – and others will involve your GP.

Foods to Eat

- **Plenty of fresh fruit and vegetables;** try to have a lot of vitamin C, which seems to lessen the symptoms of gout, easing inflammation and lowering uric acid levels.
- **In studies, it was found that drinking a glass of low-fat milk** a day can help to reduce attacks. In fact, aim for three low-fat dairy portions a day.
- **Three or four cups of coffee a day** have been shown to reduce the frequency of attacks, possibly because of a compound the coffee contains.
- **Drink plenty of water** to keep your urine a light straw colour.
- **A low-GL diet can help** reduce insulin levels.

Foods to Avoid

- **Restrict meat, fish and seafood to one portion a day because of the purines they contain.** Choose other protein sources (dairy and plant proteins). See recipe on page 191.
- **Cut down on alcohol,** particularly beer and red wine – again, because of the purines. White wine is fine in moderation.
- **Avoid fruit juice and other sugary soft drinks.** The fructose could make your gout worse.

Expert Tips

- **Gout isn't a 'stand-alone' condition;** it's an inflammatory illness that is linked to other illnesses such as cardiovascular disease, kidney stones and diabetes. It may be a good idea to take fish-oil capsules to reduce inflammation in the body, but talk to your GP rather than self-prescribing.
- **If you are overweight,** losing weight will really help.

WARNING

Your GP may prescribe anti-inflammatories. NSAIDs such as ibuprofen or indomethacin break down the gout crystals and relieve pain. Don't take them on an empty stomach, though, as that can put you at risk of gastric ulcers.

See also: Arthritis, Overweight, Kidney Stones, Diabetes

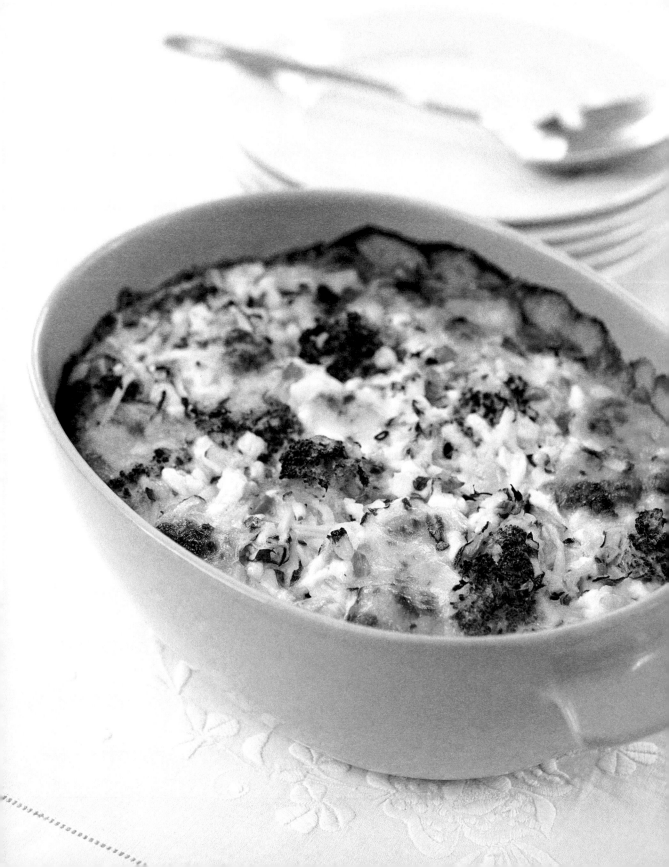

CHEESY NOODLE BAKE

Serves 4
Preparation time: 15 minutes
Cooking time: 1 hour 20 minutes

1. Preheat oven to 180°C/160°C fan/gas 4. Grease a large ovenproof dish with a little oil.

2. Fry the onion in the remaining oil over a moderate heat, covered, for 10 minutes or until soft and translucent but not browned, then add the carrot and garlic and cook for a further 5 to 6 minutes. Add the chilli and flour to the pan and cook for 2 minutes, stirring all the time. Remove from the heat and leave to cool.

3. In a pan of boiling water, blanch the broccoli florets for 1 minute, drain and refresh in cold water.

4. In a large bowl, gently whisk together the cottage cheese, eggs and milk. Carefully stir in the remaining ingredients, including the cooled onions and carrot, and season with freshly ground black pepper. Pour all of the mixture into the prepared dish and bake for one hour until golden and firm to the touch.

Ingredients

2 tablespoons rapeseed or olive oil

1 large onion, finely chopped

1 carrot, peeled and finely chopped

1 clove garlic, crushed

A pinch of chilli flakes or cayenne

3 tablespoons plain flour

1 head broccoli, cut into bite-sized florets

500g cottage cheese

3 medium eggs

150ml skimmed milk

½ courgette, coarsely grated

100g low-fat mature white cheese, cubed

½ teaspoon flat leaf parsley, finely chopped

½ teaspoon chives, finely chopped

100g medium egg noodles, cooked as per pack instructions and chilled under cold running water

Freshly ground black pepper

Per serving: 497 kcals	38g protein	23g fat	8g saturated fat	38g carbs	11g sugar	5g fibre	1.7g salt

HANGOVER

Most people know the symptoms of a hangover – feeling sick, dizzy and headachy, maybe being over-sensitive to light or loud noises, finding it hard to concentrate and even stay upright. And most people know what causes it: too much alcohol.

THE SCIENCE

Excess alcohol causes blood vessels to swell up so you get throbbing headaches and bloodshot eyes. It also causes inflammation of the stomach that makes you feel nauseous, may make you throw up and causes excess stomach acid to be produced. You might also get diarrhoea as the small bowel absorbs less water and propels the contents along. It can reduce and destabilize blood sugars, causing a feeling of exhaustion, and it also dehydrates you, causing thirst, dizziness and headache. Alcohol addiction can cause sweating, anxiety, tremors and palpitations and other side effects of withdrawal from alcohol.

The best way of dealing with a hangover is to try to prevent it from happening, so drink lots of (non-alcoholic!) fluid before you go to bed. Once a hangover's actually struck, there are some things that can help, but don't take aspirin or ibuprofen for headaches, as they can add to stomach inflammation. First, try a sports drink to rehydrate you (buy one or make your own – see below); they will be more effective than plain water. Then you need to replace all the vitamins that the excess alcohol has leached out of your body, and a healthy version of a cooked breakfast can do that.

Foods to Eat

- **Make your own rehydration drink.** Dissolve a tablespoonful of sugar and a teaspoon of salt in a pint of water.

- **Try a healthy post-hangover breakfast to replenish your stock of nutrients:** a glass of orange juice for vitamin C; a poached egg, some baked beans, a piece of wholemeal toast, tinned tomatoes – more vitamin C – and some fried mushrooms for the B vitamins. (Or see the spinach, feta and sweet potato frittata recipe on page 194.)

Foods to Avoid

- **Alcohol.** No hair of the dog; it won't help.

- **Sugary foods and drinks,** which will have too much of an unbalancing effect on your blood sugars and send them rocketing up.

Expert Tips

- **Avoid drinking on an empty stomach,** cut down on fizzy drinks (either champagne or mixers) because the alcohol from them is absorbed more quickly, and be aware that smoking at the same time as drinking will make your hangover worse (and will also increase your risk of getting throat cancer).

- **Additives in darker alcoholic** drinks may make hangovers worse.

WARNING

It can be dangerous to drive when hungover, even if your blood-alcohol levels are under the legal limit – which they probably won't be if you've only had a few hours' sleep. Are you drinking too much? Repeated hangovers could be a sign that it's time to get real about how much you drink.

See also: Alcohol dependency and problem drinking

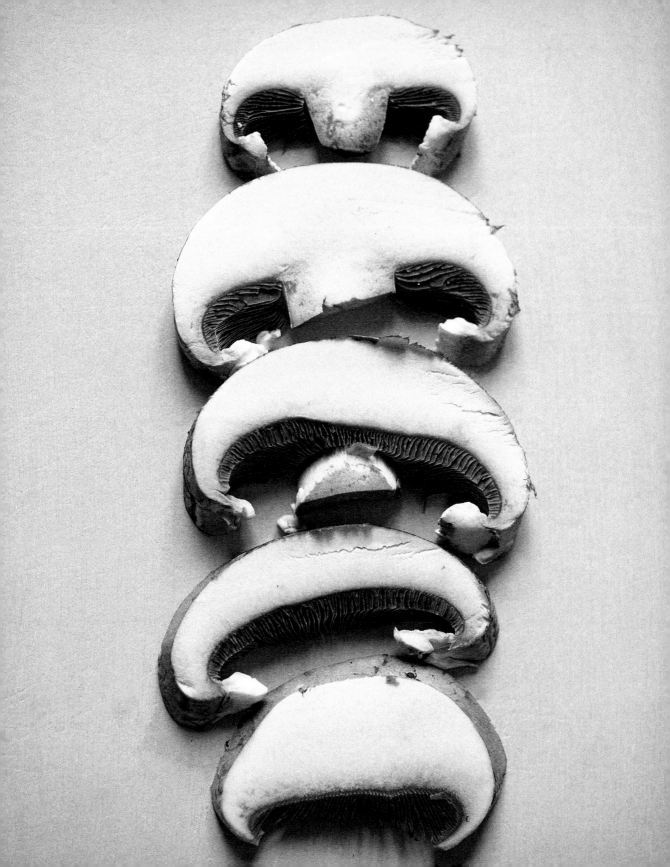

SPINACH, FETA AND SWEET POTATO FRITTATA

Serves 4
Preparation time: 5 minutes
Cooking time: 25 minutes

1. Preheat the grill to its highest setting.

2. Peel and dice the potatoes into 1cm cubes, heat 2 tablespoons of the oil in a large frying pan over a medium to high heat, and fry the sweet potatoes for 10 minutes or until tender and golden on each side. Remove from the heat while you prepare the eggs.

3. Break the eggs into a medium bowl, pour in the remaining tablespoon of oil and gently whisk. Crumble the feta into the eggs, stir in the parmesan and season with freshly ground black pepper.

4. Return the sweet potatoes to the heat, add the spinach to the pan in handfuls, stirring through each time until just wilting. Pour over the egg mixture, give the pan a quick stir to distribute the ingredients evenly, and leave to cook undisturbed for 2 to 3 minutes or until the eggs start to set.

5. Place the pan under the preheated grill for 5 minutes or until the eggs are all puffed up, golden and cooked throughout.

6. Serve warm or at room temperature for breakfast, brunch or as a light lunch with a side salad.

   You shouldn't need to add any extra salt as the feta is salty enough.

Ingredients

600g sweet potatoes
3 tablespoons olive oil
8 medium eggs
200g feta
1 tablespoon finely grated parmesan
Freshly ground black pepper
150g baby spinach

Per serving: 464 kcals	26g protein	28g fat	11g saturated fat	33g carbs	9g sugar	6g fibre	2.3g salt

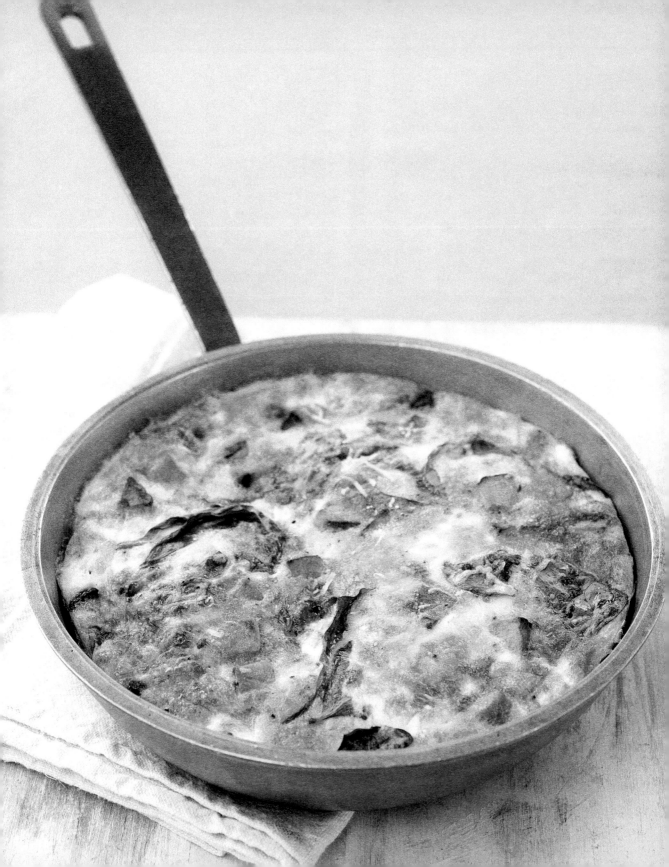

HAY FEVER

It's thought that about twenty per cent of the UK population is affected by hay fever (allergic rhinitis is the medical term) to some degree. Symptoms can include a runny nose, itchy eyes, sneezing, a cough and sinus congestion. You're more likely to get hay fever if you have other allergies such as asthma and eczema, because your immune system is over-reactive. Hay fever is more common if there's a family history of allergies, if you were exposed to cigarette smoke as a baby and if you're male. For most people, it's a spring and summer thing, but there are some unfortunates who suffer all year round. Hay fever can really interfere with your everyday life, but there are things you can do to reduce its impact.

THE SCIENCE

Basically, hay fever is an allergic reaction (and has nothing to do with hay or having a fever!). Your immune system is reacting to the presence of a substance your body has come into contact with, and is reacting as though the substance was harmful (even though it isn't). Cells in the lining of your nose, eyes and mouth release histamine, which sets off all the horrible symptoms – and your weepy eyes, runny nose and coughing are the result of your body trying to fight these harmless substances. Every single time you come into contact with them, your body reacts even more in a process called sensitization: it has become sensitized to their presence. So what can they be? There are a range of possibilities, and just because you react to one doesn't mean you'll react to the others. Plants are a common trigger, particularly pollen from grass and trees; dust mites are another, and so is pet 'residue' (saliva and skin). Spores from fungi and mould can also be problematic for some people – but pollen is the big one.

Over-the-counter antihistamines help many sufferers, but you can also get help from your GP if your hay fever is particularly bad or persistent. This can include anti-inflammatory nasal sprays and, for long-term treatment, immunotherapy: tiny, multiple injections under the skin containing minute amounts of the substances causing your allergy, given over a period of years. Your body gradually becomes used to them in a controlled way, and this lessens their effect.

On an everyday, practical level, you can also help by minimizing your exposure to whatever triggers your attacks. This doesn't mean locking yourself inside for the whole of the summer, but certain adaptations can make your life easier. For example, pollen counts are higher in the mornings, so avoid outdoor activities that could expose you to a lot of pollen at that time; wear wraparound sunglasses which can stop pollen getting in your eyes; and dust with a wet cloth rather than a dry one to collect dust rather than spread it around.

Foods to Eat

- **A Mediterranean diet** has been associated with helping hay fever symptoms, and is well worth a try. Go for whole grains, lots of fruit and vegetables, plenty of fish but not much red meat, some dairy products, olives and olive oil ...

- **There have been studies that suggest probiotic bacteria** can help modify the reaction to grass pollen, so try live yoghurt (you don't have to buy branded yoghurt drinks) and see if it works for you.

Foods to Avoid

- **Soya** allergies have been linked to hay fever, so exclude them for four weeks to see if symptoms improve, then reintroduce them to see if it gets worse again.

Expert Tip

Some people claim that eating locally produced honey relieves hay fever. There doesn't seem to be any strong scientific evidence supporting honey as an anti-allergen (it is antibacterial, though), but there's anecdotal evidence that some sufferers have experienced positive effects.

WARNING

There are lots of 'alternative' therapies for hay fever. Do be aware that some can react with other medication you are taking, so be careful and check with your GP before taking any herbal remedies.

See also: Asthma, Eczema, Sinusitis

CASE STUDY

Marie developed hay fever as a small child; every time the grass was cut outside her home she would end up with streaming eyes, sneezing uncontrollably. Tests were done to see if she reacted to anything else, and they showed up an allergy to cats. In practice, she was fine with the family cat, though meeting other people's pets could be problematic, and she dealt with the sneezing by taking antihistamines and staying inside when the grass cutters arrived. Both her parents smoked, and though the hay fever seemed to get better by itself as she got older, she went on to develop asthma – which is now fully controlled.

HEADACHE

There are many different kinds of headache. Tension headaches feel like a tight band across the front of your head at both sides. Sinus headaches are felt around the eye sockets. Cluster headaches are much rarer, though they're more common in men. These cause a pain behind the eyes, often behind one. Headaches are considered chronic when they strike on more than half the days in the month.

THE SCIENCE

Headaches are frequently related to stress and muscle tension and many sufferers have found that exercise and relaxation techniques can help. Sudden release of stress can bring about headaches, too, which is why you can get a headache when you catch up on sleep after a busy working week: levels of stress hormones drop and neurotransmitters are released rapidly. They make the blood vessels constrict and dilate – and you've got a headache. Dehydration can be another factor, as can lack of physical activity, smoking, drinking lots of coffee or alcohol, and skipping meals.

Some recent work suggests that one cause of persistent headaches may be sensitivity to artificial ingredients included in food or drink, such as the sweetener aspartame. Colas have been implicated, as well as chocolate drinks, processed meats – that's probably because of the nitrates they contain, which can dilate blood vessels – and pickles. Ice-cream headaches (caused by constriction of the blood vessels) are very common and over in a trice. Bright lights, changes in the weather and bad posture are all potential causes.

You can develop rebound headaches from using too many painkillers to treat your headaches. If you are regularly taking medication for your thumping headache, see your GP instead.

Foods to Eat

- **Keep to a healthy low-GL diet,** and remember to eat regularly. Don't let four hours go by without having a meal or snack of some kind.
- **Stay hydrated** – drink at least two litres of water a day – to avoid dehydration headaches.

Foods to Avoid

- **Caffeine intake should be low – a maximum of one coffee and two teas a day.** Avoid fizzy drinks.
- **Avoid any processed foods containing aspartame or nitrates.** You may also want to avoid icy frozen foods and drinks.

Expert Tip

- **Try keeping a trigger diary to see if any foods affect you over a couple of weeks.** If anything looks likely to be a culprit cut it out, then reintroduce it and see if your headaches start up again.

WARNING

There are some serious causes for headaches. See a doctor immediately if:

- you've had a sudden onset of a violent headache 'like a hammer on the head'
- your headache is accompanied by other signs that all is not well – including visual distrubances or a fever
- you have recently had a blow to the head.

You also need medical attention if:

- simple measures, such as taking painkillers, don't work.

See also: Migraine, Sinusitis

INFERTILITY

Infertility sounds final, but most people aren't actually infertile as such; they are 'sub-fertile'. The usual definition of infertility is an 'inability to conceive after a whole year of unprotected sex'. About eighty-five per cent of those trying will get pregnant within twelve months, and another fifty per cent overall in the next three years. Subfertility affects about fifteen per cent of couples trying to get pregnant, but there's a lot of hope for most.

THE SCIENCE

There are many different causes of infertility, affecting both men and women: endometriosis, polycystic ovaries, fibroids; erectile dysfunction, low sperm count … Both of you need to go and get checked out to find out what is going on. About twenty per cent of cases are to do with the male partner, about thirty per cent are related to both partners and the rest are female-only reasons.

Treatment will be individually tailored, depending on what the specific problem is, but there are some general lifestyle changes that will help. For men, keep your diet as healthy as possible and you won't run the risk of developing any of the deficiencies that affect the quality of your sperm. Be careful that you're not overheating your testes by wearing tight clothing or doing a lot of cycling in tight shorts, which could have that effect. Alcohol and smoking will both affect your sperm count, so limit the amount you drink and stop smoking. And men who regularly smoke marijuana are likely to have a lower sperm count and reduced fertility.

Women should eat healthily as well, and may also need to keep tabs on caffeine. There are indications that having more than a couple of coffees a day can affect your fertility. Optimizing your weight will help, especially if polycystic ovary syndrome (PCOS) is the problem. Lose some weight if you're too heavy and start doing more exercise, to get yourself in the best possible state of health for fertility. Being underweight can be just as critical: if you have a very low BMI, you may not be ovulating. That's common in anorexics, but it's also true for people who are naturally very tiny, or those who follow strict diets or are serious athletes. Make sure your overall diet is as good as it can be and that you're getting enough iron, especially if you're vegetarian or suffer from heavy periods.

Foods to Eat

- **Fresh fruit and veg,** wholegrain products and nuts keep up the levels of trace elements like selenium and zinc, as well as ensuring you get plenty of folic acid and vitamin C. They are good for all-round health for both sexes, and for healthy sperm production by men.

- **For women, make sure your diet is rich in vitamin B12 and zinc.** Meat and fish, dairy products and eggs are good sources of B12 and zinc. Take a 400mg folic acid supplement when you are trying to conceive.

- **Iron levels also need to be good.** Meat is the simplest source of iron for the body to deal with; it's also in leafy green veg like spinach, but it's not so easily processed and you have to eat a lot to get the same benefits.

Foods to Avoid

- **Alcohol.** Be sparing with booze, especially if you're male – it can have negative effects on your sperm.

- **Avoid processed food,** fast food and ready meals, because the more of these you eat, the less healthy food you're likely to fit in – and they're often high in fat or sugar, which won't help with any weight issues.

Expert Tips

- **There's another reason for watching your caffeine intake if you're female:** high levels of caffeine are associated with early miscarriages. Don't forget that caffeine isn't just in coffee: energy drinks are often just as high, and there are significant amounts in other fizzy drinks and tea as well as over-the-counter pain medications.

- **Vegetarian women can find it difficult to get enough iron;** you may need to take a supplement.

- **If you're trying to get pregnant** you should be taking folate supplement of at least 400mcg a day.

WARNING

It can be tempting to try anything when you're desperate, and that can include all sorts of experimental procedures in private clinics. It's sometimes difficult to know what's controversial and what isn't, but read widely on the subject, because some treatments can be ruinously expensive and still not give you the baby you crave.

See also: Endometriosis, Erectile dysfunction, Obesity and being overweight, Polycystic ovaries

INFLUENZA

Influenza is highly infectious and, unlike the common cold, it can be a killer. Take it seriously, especially if you have any chronic conditions such as diabetes, asthma, chronic chest diseases or problems with your immune system – or if you are old or very young. Symptoms of flu include a temperature that suddenly shoots up to more than 38°C, and extreme fatigue. Your joints and muscles will probably ache a lot, and you may feel sick and dizzy. Go to bed, keep warm, take paracetamol-based cold remedies and drink plenty of liquids, and you should be fine after a few days if you were reasonably fit and well to start with. Just stay inside and minimize your contact with the outside world, to avoid infecting other people who may not be able to fight it off so easily.

THE SCIENCE

Flu is caused by a virus, just like coughs and colds, so antibiotics won't cure it. It is, however, more likely to cause complications than colds and coughs, particularly secondary chest infections. Bacteria can grow in the lungs as they are already weakened because of the virus. If you fall into one of the high-risk groups, your GP may prescribe drugs such as oseltamivir (i.e. Tamiflu) to help reduce the length of your flu (but this needs to be taken within the first few days to be most effective).

Flu is spread just like colds, via droplets sneezed or coughed into the air by somebody who already has the virus, and it can also spread by touch. The symptoms will develop a couple of days after you've been infected, and you will be infectious just before your symptoms become obvious, and for the following five to six days. The flu virus changes every year, and having an annual flu jab is the most useful thing you can do when it comes to preventing it. Keep fit, and help your immune system to fight off flu by making sure your diet is as healthy as it can be.

Foods to Eat

- **Lots of fruits and vegetables** will boost your immune system and can help fight off flu or lower the risk of it hitting you. To get the maximum nutrients, eat fruit and veg in as wide a range of colours as possible: red tomatoes and peppers, green leafy veg, dark blueberries and plums, yellow peaches and nectarines.
- **Drink lots of water;** it's important to keep hydrated.

Foods to Avoid

- **Dairy products, particularly milk,** can sometimes increase mucus production, so choose a calcium-enriched milk substitute while you are ill.

Expert Tips

- **You're unlikely to feel much like food when you're in the throes of flu,** but keep ingredients to hand so you can eat when you feel like it. As you get better, try home-made chicken soup – a traditional remedy that's supposed to boost your immune system (see page 176).
- **During the flu season,** take particular care to wash your hands whenever you have been in public places.

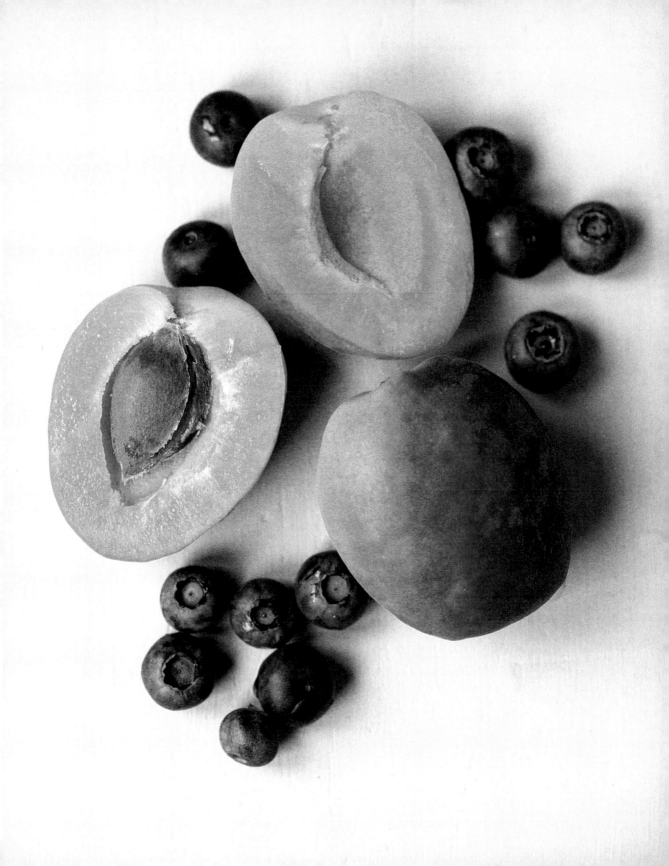

MIGRAINE

People who suffer from migraine – disabling, one-sided, violent headaches – have a horrible time. They may have disturbed vision with flashes of light, feel and be sick, even lose some sensation in an arm or feel it tingling. Migraines are much more than ordinary headaches, and have been described as the 'most common neurological condition' around. There's no cure as such, but migraines can be controlled. Different things work for different people, so try a few. Action is always better than waiting for the next migraine to strike!

THE SCIENCE

Migraines are thought to be linked to levels of serotonin in the brain. Low levels make blood vessels constrict in a particular area (that's what is thought to cause the visual disturbances and numbness), and they then dilate (causing the headache), but exactly what makes this happen is not understood.

What is known is that some people's migraines are prompted by triggers: substances or circumstances that can provoke an attack. Hormones can be involved; migraines are more common in women than men, and they may get worse with pregnancy, periods or puberty. These migraines seem to be related to oestrogens, so if you're suffering from frequent migraines and taking a combined contraceptive pill, you may be advised to change. Stress can be a factor – both emotional and physical stress. Some migraine sufferers can identify environmental triggers, such as people smoking nearby or flickering lighting, while others find that attacks are provoked by what they eat or drink (either specific foods, or simply missing meals).

Don't be disheartened if you fail to identify a trigger; only about thirty per cent of migraine sufferers do. To see if you fall into that thirty per cent, you need to keep a detailed symptom and trigger diary over a period of time, and remember to include external circumstances as well as foods you suspect of being involved – stressful situations, perhaps, or even weather conditions. You might see a clear pattern emerge. If that's the case, then remove that trigger as far as it's possible and see if your migraines improve in frequency or intensity. Next, you need to rule out the possibility of coincidence, so you should reintroduce it and see what happens. It's worth doing that double-check, unpleasant though the consequences might be. Don't get fixated on finding a trigger – there may not be one for you to uncover.

All migraines are different to some degree, and you may have to experiment before you find a combination of treatments that works for you. Talk to your GP or pharmacist about the medications you can try and learn to spot warning signs, because painkillers are most effective if you take them before the headache really hits. Lying in a darkened room is often the best thing to do, and holding cool cloths to your head might help.

Foods high in vitamin B2 (riboflavin) are said to help migraine sufferers: eggs, fish, dairy products such as yoghurt and cottage cheese.

Magnesium deficiency can contribute to migraines, so make sure there's plenty in your diet. Eat whole grains and avoid refined products; have plenty of vegetables and pulses (see recipe on page 206), and it's worth noting that soya is a good source of magnesium – try a stir-fry with tofu, perhaps, or a soya yoghurt.

Drink plenty of water, especially during an attack.

The most common triggers seem to be red wine, chocolate and caffeine. Try cutting those out one by one. If they don't make a difference, try spices, nuts and seeds, seafood, starches and food additives. All of these are reported migraine triggers.

The flavour enhancer MSG is another frequent trigger. It's often in ready meals and fast food, especially Chinese food, so stick to dishes you prepare and cook yourself, and see what happens to your migraines (that would also remove other possibly troublesome flavourings and colorants from your diet – things that manufacturers use but home cooks do not).

Another reason for cutting caffeine is that it can be dehydrating, and you need to stay hydrated. Try swapping your coffee and tea for herb or fruit teas (but not dandelion tea, which has a diuretic effect).

WARNING

Some dangerous conditions can cause pain in the eyes and visual disturbances (glaucoma, for example, after middle age), so don't automatically assume that it's migraine; see your GP.

If you are pregnant or breastfeeding, migraine medications can be dangerous. Headaches and visual disturbance in pregnancy can be a sign of pre-eclampsia, so see a doctor immediately.

See also: Headache

HUMMUS AND SALSA SNACK

Serves 6
Preparation time: 15 minutes

1. To make the hummus, tip the chickpeas into the bowl of a food processor along with the water, tahini, lemon juice, olive oil and cumin, and blend until you reach your desired consistency. If it is a little thick add a little more water. Season to taste with a little sea salt and freshly ground pepper. Spoon into a small serving bowl and sprinkle with the paprika.

2. To make the salsa, combine all of the ingredients in a small bowl, season to taste with sea salt and freshly ground black pepper.

3. Serve both dips with a mixture of breadsticks, crackers and/or crudités.

Ingredients

Hummus

400g tinned chickpeas, rinsed and drained

100ml water

4 tablespoons tahini

Juice of 1 lemon

1½ tablespoons extra virgin olive oil

1 teaspoon ground cumin

¼ teaspoon smoked paprika

Sea salt and freshly ground black pepper

Salsa

5 plum tomatoes, finely diced

½ red onion, finely chopped

2 cloves garlic, crushed

1 red or green chilli, deseeded and finely diced

1 tablespoon coriander, finely chopped

To serve

Wholegrain breadsticks

Wholegrain crackers

Vegetable crudités, eg. carrots, cucumber, celery

| Per serving: 150 kcals | 5.5g protein | 10g fat | 1.5g saturated fat | 10g carbs | 3.1g sugar | 4.5g fibre | 0.26g salt |

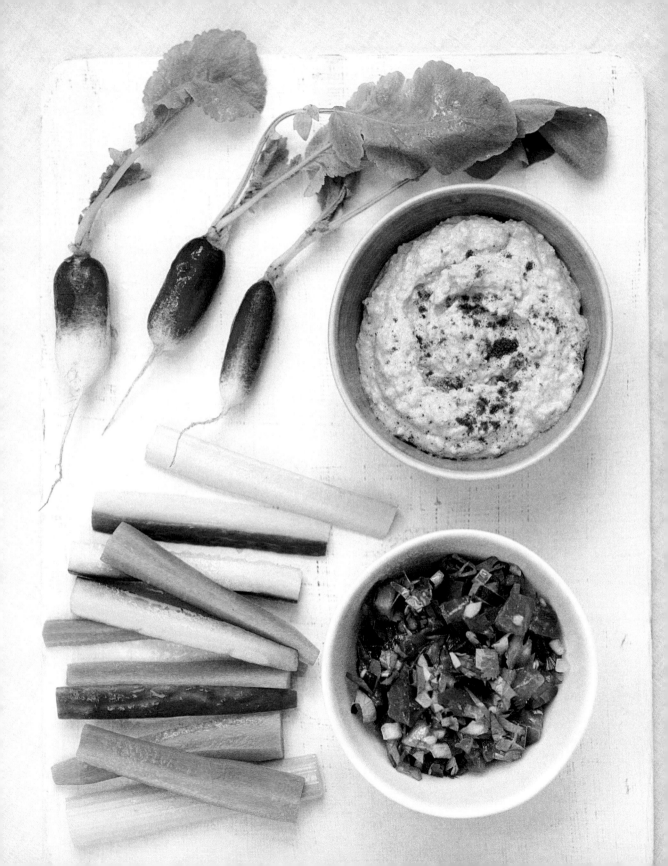

RESTLESS LEGS

If your legs often feel uncomfortable, twitchy or prickly when you're resting and you have to move them about to get some relief, you may be suffering from Restless Leg Syndrome, or RLS. They might even be keeping you awake, possibly jerking involuntarily at night. This is fairly common, and it's twice as likely in women as in men.

THE SCIENCE

The exact causes of RLS are unknown, though there's some evidence that it's related to the levels of dopamine, a chemical neurotransmitter in the brain. One type – secondary RLS – is connected to other conditions and can also occur during pregnancy (if they're pregnancy-related, then RLS symptoms will die down naturally in time).

Your GP may refer you for blood tests to check whether there are any underlying conditions that can explain your twitchy legs, and if yours are severe you may also have muscle function and sleep tests. If there's anything behind your RLS it can be treated appropriately. There's also a lot you can do yourself. Firstly, if you're a smoker, stop, as this can affect the blood supply to the legs. Initial studies have shown that taking some regular exercise during the day makes a difference, but avoid this just before bedtime. If you have problems sleeping at night, stick to a regular sleeping pattern and avoid naps during the day. Some people find a hot bath helps RLS, while others recommend massage. Drugs are available, but lifestyle changes are definitely worth trying first.

Foods to Eat

- **Magnesium can also help.** Nuts are a good source, and so are whole grains, beans and pulses, sunflower and sesame seeds.
- **Vitamin B complex is useful for conditions involving nerve transmission,** so make sure you're getting enough from meat, fish, whole grains and pulses.

Foods to Avoid

- **Coffee, tea and alcohol are all stimulants,** which could exacerbate the problem.

Expert Tip

- **Stretching the leg muscles can bring immediate relief,** as can bouncing the legs up and down while sitting in a chair, with the balls of the feet on the floor.

WARNING

If you have symptoms suggestive of RLS see your doctor to rule out any serious causes

See also: Anaemia, Diabetes, Insomnia

RICKETS

Rickets affects children – the adult equivalent is *osteomalacia* – and is characterized by bones that are soft and weak. It was thought it had largely died out in the UK, but in late 2010, twenty per cent of children tested for bone problems in Southampton showed signs of having rickets. The soft, weak bones of rickets can lead to poor growth, bone and muscle pain, weak muscles, and an increased risk of fractures. If it's severe or treated late, it can mean permanent deformity. This particularly affects the legs, which can become badly bowed, but it can also lead to curvature of the spine. However, if rickets is treated promptly, the outlook is very good.

THE SCIENCE

Calcium gives bones their strength, and the way the body builds bones and uses calcium is regulated by vitamin D. Children with rickets don't have enough calcium in their bones, but the problem is usually a lack of vitamin D.

Most of the vitamin D the body needs is made by the action of sunlight on the skin, so anybody who stays inside a lot or who covers up when they go out might be lacking in vitamin D. It's more of a problem – not surprisingly – in cold countries, but people with dark skin can also suffer from a lack of vitamin D. Any child who doesn't go outside much is potentially at risk. If you're a woman with low vitamin D levels and you're breastfeeding, then your baby won't be getting enough vitamin D from your milk, and that can cause rickets. The other source of vitamin D is food, so make sure that you and your family are eating a healthy diet; one which contains enough calcium as well. Rickets is treated by supplements (or an annual injection), but it's important to make dietary and lifestyle changes too.

Foods to Eat

- **Oily fish, liver, cheese, butter and eggs will boost your vitamin D levels,** as will fortified breakfast cereals and spreads.
- **Dairy products – milk, yoghurt, cheese – are a great source of calcium.** Tinned salmon and sardines are also good if you crunch the bones. Dried fruit and sesame seeds (found in tahini) are full of calcium.

Foods to Avoid

- **Cut down on processed food and ready meals** because you need the maximum nutritional benefits from what you eat.

Expert Tips

- **If you're vegetarian or vegan, you may need to take a supplement**.
- **If you're pregnant or breastfeeding,** take a vitamin D supplement of 10mcg a day, especially if you're in a high-risk group.

WARNING

Sunlight is important but be aware of the consequences of too much sun. The official guideline is fifteen minutes on your hands and face a few times a week during spring and summer.

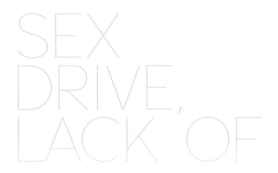

SEX DRIVE, LACK OF

Sex drive – libido – is completely individual, and the important thing is to recognize what's normal for you. Everyone's expectations are different, and it's only a problem if it's damaging your relationship or making you unhappy. It can be important to recognize that there are other factors that can affect your libido and that low libido may not reflect your feelings for your partner.

THE SCIENCE

There are many reasons why people go off the idea of sex. It can be situational and just affect you at particular times; maybe you're not a morning person, or perhaps a new baby is taking every last ounce of energy. It's quite normal for men to experience a gradual loss of sexual interest in their partner over time and for women to do so around the menopause; but again, this varies hugely. Losing your libido can also be part of an underlying problem, such as depression, long-term stress or anxiety: all of these can affect your interest in sex. Body image – how you see yourself – can be implicated, as can low self-esteem. But some physical problems, such as

underactive thyroid and Cushing's disease, can cause a low sex drive, so talk to your doctor once you've recognized that there is a problem so he or she can rule those out.

One of the best things you can do for your libido is to take good care of yourself. If you suffer from depression or low self-esteem it's easy to let this one drift, but looking after your body will help you feel better all round. Keep your diet as healthy as possible. Aphrodisiacs – chocolate, oysters, asparagus, even champagne – are unlikely to have any major physical effects but may help you psychologically.

Foods to Eat

- **Make sure you get enough micronutrients:** lots of fresh fruit and vegetables, lean meat, fish and seafood, eggs, low-fat dairy products, some nuts and seeds, whole grains. The better your diet, the better you'll feel about yourself.
- **Your body needs zinc to make sex hormones,** and you can find plenty of websites suggesting that taking zinc will improve your libido. In fact, the link – if there is one – is more tenuous than that. Eat healthily, especially seafood, and you'll have enough zinc in your diet anyway.

Foods to Avoid

- **Alcohol in excess can definitely reduce your libido,** and so can street drugs.
- **Fast food and processed food that's high in salt, fat and sugar but low in nutrients** can have negative effects.

Expert Tip

- **There is no such thing as the male menopause,** although it is normal for testosterone levels to decline with age. Testosterone supplementation is controversial: it may be beneficial but may also carry serious health risks.

SINUSITIS

If you've pain and tenderness around your eyes, cheekbones, forehead and beside your nose, you may well have sinusitis. Bend or move your head around: it will probably get worse, and turn into a throbbing pain. You may lose your sense of smell, develop a runny or blocked nose, have a pain in your jaw, and a temperature! It's all rather debilitating, but about two-thirds of sinusitis cases clear up by themselves within about three weeks.

THE SCIENCE

The front of the skull contains cavities which are usually full of air, and are lined with soft tissue. During an attack of sinusitis the tissue becomes inflamed and produces mucus, as a result of a viral infection such as a cold. This prevents the normal drainage of the cavities and blocks them up. Steaming – bending your head over a bowl of hot water and using a towel to cover both your head and the bowl, then breathing in for a few minutes – can help clear the mucus, but be careful you don't burn yourself. Sleeping with your head raised on an extra pillow or two can help, as can a humidifier.

Chronic sinusitis is often caused by allergies (like hay fever) which provoke excess production of mucus. Sometimes the tissue lining the sinuses develops small polyps, harmless growths like skin tags, which produce more mucus. These can be surgically removed if they become troublesome. Treatments for chronic sinusitis include anti-inflammatory nasal sprays, decongestants and sometimes antibiotics; talk to your GP if your sinusitis lasts a long time or keeps recurring.

Foods to Eat

- **Fruit and vegetables, wholegrain carbs and very little saturated fat** to boost your immune system.
- **Drink plenty of fluids,** especially water.

Foods to Avoid

- **Cut the caffeine and alcohol** – they are dehydrating. Remember that many fizzy drinks contain large amounts of caffeine, particularly colas.
- **Some people report that dairy products make their sinusitis worse** by increasing the amount of mucus produced. It doesn't seem to make a difference for others. Don't remove all dairy from your diet long-term without taking steps to ensure you get enough calcium from other foods.

Expert Tips

- **Avoid smoky environments,** which can aggravate sinusitis.
- **Some people swear by rinsing out their sinuses with salt water** to clear mucus secretions, but this can take a bit of practice to perfect.
- **Add eucalyptus or menthol oil to the boiling water** you use to inhale steam from.

WARNING

If a child is the one showing signs of sinusitis, go to your GP; there can be complications in children that need to be ruled out.

See also: Colds and coughs, Headaches, Asthma, Hay fever

SNORING

Everyone knows what snoring is – it's the racket someone else produces that stops you from going to sleep! There are different degrees of snoring, from simple snuffling noises right through to the deafening snoring caused by sleep apnoea, and it can have pernicious effects, on both you and the people around you, so it is worth seeking help.

THE SCIENCE

Snoring is caused when the muscles and tissues at the back of the throat relax during deep sleep and partially block the airway. Air has to be pushed past the blockage, and that causes the tissues and tongue to vibrate. It doesn't help if you're overweight (a big cause of snoring is obesity) or have a chronically blocked nose, as the airway is already narrowed. Nasal strips can help to relieve congestion, as can trying not to sleep on your back. Alcohol can also be a factor because it is a depressant and causes further sedation.

Sleep apnoea takes snoring to a new level; the airway is almost completely blocked when you're asleep. A classic sign is that a partner will notice uncomfortably long pauses between breaths – literally, they stop breathing. As a result, the level of oxygen in the blood goes right down and carbon dioxide levels go right up, so much so that your body is alerted to this dangerous state of affairs and wakes you up so that you can breathe. Your sleep can be interrupted all night, resulting in chronic fatigue.

Sleep apnoea can be diagnosed and treated; you may have to undergo formal sleep studies and possibly surgery, which may sound daunting – but don't dismiss it as 'just bad snoring', because it can be life-threatening.

Foods to Eat

Keep your weight within a healthy range and eat a varied, balanced diet. Swap refined foods for wholegrain versions, eat lots of vegetables and have fruit instead of sweets.

Foods to Avoid

Don't drink alcohol if you have a serious snoring problem, not just because of the congeners, but also because it makes your muscles relax and block the airway more than they normally would.

Cut out fatty foods like chips; avoid processed food, fast food and ready meals.

Expert Tips

Sleeping tablets can make snoring worse, so try to avoid them.

Stop smoking – it definitely makes snoring worse.

WARNING

Untreated sleep apnoea causes long-term health risks. See a doctor if you wake up during the night because you can't breath, or if your partner reports loud snoring followed by a long silence. It's also a good idea to get medical advice if your snoring is ruining your relationship.

See also: Colds and coughs, Chronic fatigue syndrome, Insomnia, Obesity and Weight

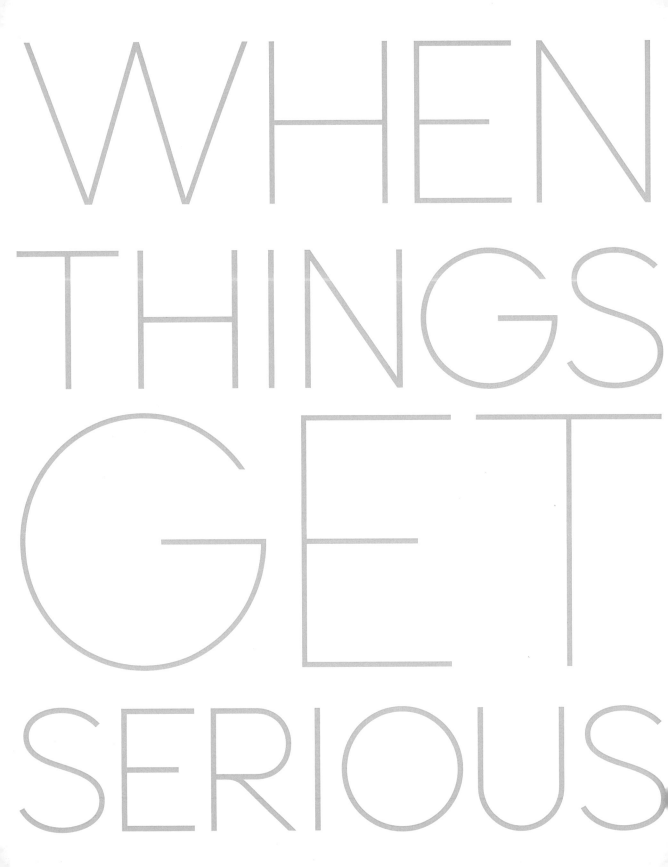

WHEN THINGS GET SERIOUS

If one or both of your parents died prematurely of heart disease, stroke or cancer, you should be taking steps to protect yourself unless you want to follow in their footsteps. That means eating a healthy diet, exercising regularly, not smoking, sticking within the government's alcohol recommendations and keeping your weight under control. The sooner you start, the better. Don't wait for the warning signs that things are starting to go wrong, such as high cholesterol levels showing up in blood tests, or a diagnosis of Type 2 diabetes. Even if you don't have a family history of premature death, it's worth leading as healthy a life as you can, to ensure that you are not the one to break the pattern!

If you already have a serious chronic health condition, the more you learn about it, the better able you will be to deal with it. There have been many scientific trials in recent years about the ways in which nutrition can alleviate the symptoms caused by major diseases, and even reverse some of the damage done to the body. We've included some of the most exciting findings in these pages, but you should consult your doctor or specialist before adopting any new diet, just in case there are contraindications to it in your particular case. Think of these recommendations as a topic for discussion rather than a hard-and-fast prescription.

It's crucial that you don't try to self-diagnose or self-treat any of the conditions described in this section. If you have any significant symptoms that make you feel unwell for more than a few days, you should see your doctor, who will be able to decide whether any of them require further investigation and treatment.

ANAEMIA

Red blood cells carry oxygen around the body, and anaemia occurs when we don't have enough of them. The primary symptom of anaemia is tiredness. If you're anaemic, you may have to drag yourself out of bed in the morning and you could frequently find yourself feeling exhausted during the day. When you exercise, you run out of energy quickly and may find that your legs feel leaden. You could experience dizziness on standing up, headaches, palpitations, fluttery heart and shortness of breath, and your complexion may be very pale. Your GP will refer you for a full blood count test, which will confirm whether or not you are anaemic. (There are many other causes of feeling tired which may also need to be looked into.)

THE SCIENCE

Bone marrow produces our red blood cells and other components of blood, and it does so at a very rapid rate, making millions of them a day. The fast production consumes a great number of vitamins and micronutrients, so clearly any deficiency in your diet can quite rapidly translate into anaemia. The principal nutrients required by the bone marrow for making red blood cells are iron, vitamin B12 and folate, so it's essential that we get enough of them in our diets.

A number of inherited conditions, such as sickle cell disease and thalassemia, cause faster turnover of blood cells than normal, so sufferers are more sensitive to nutritional deficiencies. Women with heavy periods lose a lot of iron, and vegetarians and vegans may also get iron deficiency unless they keep a careful eye on their intake. Pernicious anaemia is caused by an auto-immune condition in which your immune system attacks the mechanism that allows you to absorb B12 properly. So no matter how much you take by mouth, you can't absorb it. People with this condition require injections to maintain their B12 levels, or they take tablets that are absorbed under the tongue.

Once anaemia is diagnosed, it's important to pinpoint the cause because, very rarely, it could be something serious such as leukaemia (affecting the bone marrow), or internal bleeding (from a cancer). Once the cause is known, your doctor will want to address it as well as giving you medication to make up the deficiency.

For iron deficiency, you will be given ferrous sulphate. Take the pills first thing in the morning with a glass of orange juice, because iron needs vitamin C to aid its absorption in the digestive system. Don't drink tea or coffee or any calcium-containing foods for at least half an hour afterwards, because these can all impair the absorption of iron. For folate deficiency, you will be given folic acid tablets.

Addressing your diet can help to make up any deficiencies, so increase your dietary intake of the nutrient you are lacking – but follow your doctor's instructions as well.

Foods to Eat

- **For iron,** eat more red meat (especially liver and kidneys – see recipe on page 218), chicken, oily fish, whole grains and eggs. Iron from animal sources is more easily absorbed and you don't need to combine it with vitamin C to aid absorption. Some dried fruits, especially dried apricots, are good sources of iron, as are dark green leafy vegetables – but don't overcook them or the iron content with be lost.
- **For vitamin B12,** eat meat, fish, eggs, cheese, and if you are vegetarian look for breakfast cereals, milks and spreads that are fortified with B12 (also known as cobalamin).
- **You'll find folate** in green vegetables, nuts and wholegrain products.

Foods to Avoid

- **Don't take any form of caffeine or anything containing calcium** within half an hour of taking an iron supplement or you won't absorb it properly.
- **Antacids,** taken for indigestion, can affect the absorption of iron.

Expert Tips

- **Keep exercising but don't overdo it** when you are anaemic as you could get breathless and put a strain on your heart.
- **Pregnancy can cause a 'natural' anaemia.** It's important to go for all the blood tests you are offered to detect a low blood count, because it could cause complications.

WARNING

Severe iron-deficiency anaemia can cause heart failure, when your heart is no longer able to pump enough blood around your body to supply the major organs, so if you are told by your doctor to take iron tablets, make sure you take them.

CASE STUDY

Jane had heavy periods throughout her forties that left her feeling drained and exhausted. A blood test found that she had iron-deficiency anaemia and her doctor told her to take ferrous sulphate tablets. If her blood counts didn't go up within three weeks, she was told she would need a blood transfusion. The tablets made her feel nauseous and caused constipation, so she stuck to the lowest dose she could, but began to focus on eating iron-rich foods at every meal as well. She was told that black-strap molasses were a particularly rich source, so she took a couple of spoonfuls a day. Fortunately, her blood counts went up enough to avoid the transfusion, and once they were at a normal level, she was able to stop taking the tablets. From then on, after every period she would eat liver, spinach, lentils and blackstrap molasses to make up any deficiency the bleeding might have caused.

WARM SALAD OF CHICKEN LIVERS WITH APPLE AND WALNUTS

Serves 4 as a light lunch or a starter
Preparation time: 10 minutes
Cooking time: 10 minutes

Ingredients

1. Blanch the green beans in boiling water for 2 to 3 minutes, drain and refresh under plenty of cold running water, then drain well.

2. Pile the salad leaves into a large bowl or platter, add the red onion, walnuts, beans and apple, toss to distribute the ingredients evenly.

3. Heat a large frying pan over a high heat, toss the chicken livers in the oil and tip into the hot pan, cooking for 2 to 3 minutes on each side or until just browned. Remove the chicken livers from the pan, set aside and add the balsamic to the oil and leave to bubble for 30 seconds. Spoon the livers and dressing over the salad and serve.

150g green beans, trimmed

100g baby spinach leaves

100g watercress

½ red onion, thinly sliced

40g walnuts, roughly chopped

1 small green apple, cored and thinly sliced

250g chicken livers, trimmed and halved lengthwise

2 teaspoons olive oil

3 tablespoons balsamic vinegar

| Per serving: 171 kcals | 13g protein | 10g fat | 1.5g saturated fat | 7.4g carbs | 6.5g sugar | 3.5g fibre | 0.22g salt |

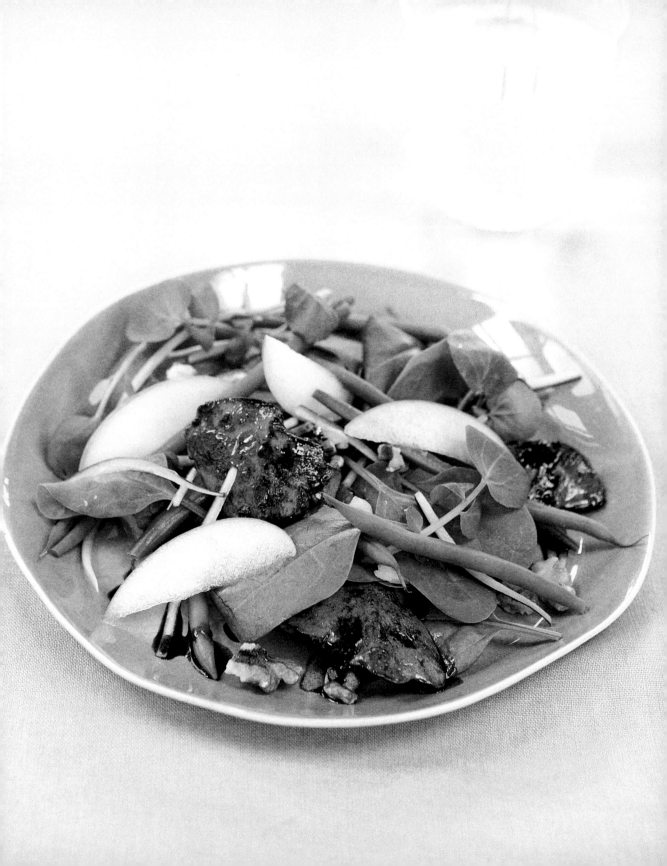

ARTHRITIS

Arthritis means 'inflammation of the joints'. The two common types – osteo- and rheumatoid – have completely different causes and treatments. Both affect the joints, though. And both can be very painful and debilitating.

OSTEOARTHRITIS

Osteoarthritis is generally just the wear and tear on joints associated with normal life. Some people's joints wear out faster than others, due to a combination of how their cartilage is constructed and how much stress they have put on their joints. If you have been a lifelong hill runner, your joints will likely wear out faster than someone who does more gentle forms of exercise, such as swimming or cycling. Being overweight for years puts extra strain on the knees and hips and is a major cause. Degeneration tends to start in the big joints, such as the knees and hips, and sufferers may eventually need replacement joints, which are good but never quite as effective as the original ones!

The symptoms of osteoarthritis can be limited if you have healthy cartilage on the ends of your bones and you don't wear it out. Managing your weight is crucial. Keeping your muscles strong by doing gentle exercise that doesn't stress the joints will help their stability and longevity. Glucosamine supplements are thought to help keep cartilage healthy in some people (try taking 1500mg a day for six weeks), and there is loads of dietary advice for anyone who is worried about joint problems.

Foods to Eat

- **Avocado soybean unsaponifiables have been shown in studies to decrease the pain and inflammation of joint problems.** These are supplements made of one third avocado oil and two thirds soybean oils. In trials, osteoarthritis sufferers who took 300mg supplements needed less pain medication, although it took two months before any effects were seen.

- **The anti-inflammatory action of oily fish can help.** Increase the number of portions you eat to two or three a week.

- **Antioxidant vitamins are very important because free radicals may have a role in the development of osteoarthritis.** Eat foods containing vitamins A (dark green and yellow fruits and veg, liver, milk, butter, cheese, eggs), C (fresh fruits and veg of all colours, such as citrus fruits, kiwi, peppers, broccoli) and E (wheatgerm, corn oil, avocados).

- **Low vitamin D levels can be associated with osteoarthritis.** Make sure you get adequate dietary sources (from fatty fish and dairy sources) and get out in the sunshine regularly.

- **Deficiency of folate and vitamin B12 can increase your risk of joint degeneration,** so keep eating organ meats, dairy products, salmon, sardines and dark green leafy veg.

- **Selenium is also important because it helps to protect the joints from oxidative stress.** Brazil nuts are the best dietary source.

RHEUMATOID ARTHRITIS

This is an immune-related condition in which, for reasons we don't quite understand, your body reacts to components within your joints in such a way that it sets up a destructive inflammation in the joint cavity, eroding the cartilage. It typically affects the hands and wrists first, but can attack any joints around the body. Treatment is aimed at reducing your body's reactivity to the inflammatory process by reducing the immune reaction. Treatments range from simple anti-inflammatories such as ibuprofen through to steroids, either in tablet form or very occasionally injected straight into the joint. You might also be prescribed immunosuppressant drugs similar to the ones given to organ transplant patients, and a particularly damaged joint might be replaced. Unlike osteoarthritis, rheumatoid arthritits can sometimes affect other organs of the body, such as the lungs and eyes, and this may need to be monitored and investigated further.

It's been found that people with rheumatoid arthritis consume more saturated fat and less fibre than average, and they often have deficiencies of micronutrients such as folate, B6, vitamin E, calcium, magnesium, copper and selenium. This may be because their impaired movement makes it difficult for them to buy and cook healthy food for themselves. It could be that depression plays a part. But some of the drugs they may be prescribed can cause them to secrete micronutrients in urine, so it's important to eat a varied, healthy diet. With poor dietary habits on top of decreased mobility, sufferers are at risk of obesity, which will only make their arthritis worse.

Foods to Eat

- **You may be recommended to take a fish oil supplement of 15ml a day.** This is an amount that it wouldn't be practical to get from food, but there's quite a lot of evidence that it can relieve the symptoms of rheumatoid arthritis.

- **Sufferers are at risk of osteoporosis,** so need to make sure they get adequate calcium and vitamin D in their diets.

- **There's an increased risk of iron deficiency because haemoglobin production is suppressed during inflammatory stages of the illness.** Keep up your dietary intake (from meat, whole grains, eggs, dried fruit and green vegetables).

- **Sufficient levels of vitamins C and E and selenium are important to counter free radical damage.** Get plenty of fruits and veg, and nibble Brazil nuts as a snack.

Foods to Avoid

- **Reduce your intake of saturated fats and 'empty' calories** – foods that have little or no nutritional benefits.

Expert Tip

- **For both types of arthritis, weight control is crucial.** The more weight the affected joints have to support, the faster they will degenerate.

WARNING

If any of your joints are unexpectely painful or tender with reduced mobility and swelling, see your doctor immediately.

See also: Depression, Osteoporosis, Obesity and being overweight

ASTHMA

More people are being diagnosed with asthma nowadays than a few decades ago. It could be due to an increase in atmospheric pollutants, such as car exhaust fumes, or because there are more allergens in our environment that cause allergic reactions, but whatever the reason it's an alarming trend because asthma can be a serious and life-threatening condition. At least one in eleven children is currently diagnosed as asthmatic, and although some of them will grow out of it, the others will continue to have the disease in adulthood. Some people will only develop asthma as adults.

THE SCIENCE

During an asthma attack, an inflammatory response in the lungs causes the airways to narrow and produce mucus. The airways of the lungs go into spasm and the sufferer will gasp for breath. There's a characteristic wheezing sound that asthmatics make as they struggle to expel air from the narrowed airways of their lungs. They might also have a persistent dry cough and feel a tightness in the chest. There's a wide spectrum of severity. Some people need regular use of a ventilator to open up the airways, while others just need to use an inhaler from time to time, for example before or during exercise.

Asthma is more common among smokers, or those who are regularly exposed to cigarette smoke. It's more common in babies with a low birth weight and in overweight adults, and people who get other immune-related disorders such as eczema, hay fever and allergies can be more prone to it.

House dust mites are a common asthma trigger. If this is the case, you will need to lift carpets and install hardwood flooring, cover your mattress in a rubberized hypoallergenic sheet and vacuum regularly to remove any dust mites and their eggs from your home environment. Cold air can be a trigger, in which case it might help to cover your nose and mouth with a scarf when you go outdoors in winter. Animal hair is another trigger, as is cigarette smoke. If symptoms occur only during the summer months, pollen could be triggering them. And exercise can sometimes bring on an attack. Asthma can get worse if you have a cold or chest infection, so needs to be treated more aggressively at these times.

Foods to Eat

- **Foods rich in omega 3s can reduce the inflammation of the lungs.** That means oily fish, such as salmon, herring and mackerel (see recipe on page 224) – unfortunately not the kinds of fish children tend to like! Omega 3s are also found in olive oil, flaxseeds and walnuts.

- **The typical Mediterranean diet has recently been associated with an improvement in the symptoms of asthmatic children.** One study showed a reduction in attacks of seventy per cent in people who were not taking medication. Mediterranean diet foods include olive oil, whole grains, tomatoes, fish, plenty of fruit and veg and only a little meat.

- **Eat plenty of foods containing vitamins C, D and E,** which can reduce the inflammation in the lungs associated with asthma.
- **Some studies have linked asthma with low dietary levels of selenium, magnesium or vitamin B6.** Include plenty of foods in your diet that contain them: Brazil nuts, whole grains, eggs, dairy products, green vegetables, meat, fish and bananas.

Foods to Avoid

- **It can be worth keeping a food and symptoms diary to see if any particular foods tend to trigger attacks.** Wheat, eggs, nuts and dairy can be culprits, but only omit them from a child's diet under the supervision of a professional dietitian.
- **Sulphites, added to food as a preservative, can trigger asthma attacks in some people.** You'll find them in some dried fruits, biscuits, snacks, fruit drinks, breakfast cereals and all kinds of processed foods. Read labels carefully and avoid anything containing E numbers 220 to 228 inclusive.
- **Limit alcohol and spicy foods that make you produce more acid,** because these cause heartburn, which can make asthma worse.
- **Cut down on saturated fats in the diet,** as these can make lung inflammation worse.

Expert Tips

- **Maintain a healthy weight and keep yourself as well as possible** so your immune system is not over-stretched.
- **Exercise as much as you can without triggering an attack,** to improve your cardiovascular fitness.
- **Smoking not only brings on asthma attacks but it also reduces the effectiveness of asthma medications.** It's truly crazy to smoke if you have asthma!
- **Asthmatics should get the flu vaccine every year** to protect themselves from the worst of the winter viruses.

CASE STUDY

Derek had mild asthma from the age of nine. At seventeen years old, he played a lot of sport and would only treat his asthma with an inhaler if it got bad when he played football. Over the winter one year it got a lot worse and he ended up in A&E with an asthma attack that he couldn't relieve with his usual inhaler. He went back to his GP, who recommended that he use a different inhaler on a daily basis, whether he had symptoms or not. His doctor suggested he install hardwood floors in his bedroom and vacuum them daily. He also suggested avoiding sulphites in foods such as dried fruit, as this could be a trigger, but encouraged him to eat fresh foods with plenty of vitamins D, C and E. Derek's symptoms improved considerably and he found he could play sport for a lot longer without experiencing any symptoms of his asthma.

WARNING

If someone's lips go blue during an asthma attack or they have difficulty completing a sentence in one breath, it means the level of oxygen in their blood is dangerously low. Call an ambulance. If possible, find an inhaler or nebulizer while waiting for the ambulance. Without treatment, such attacks can be fatal.

See also: Heartburn, Eczema

WHOLEGRAIN KEDGEREE

Serves 4
Preparation time: 15 minutes
Cooking time: 30 minutes

1. Pour the oil into a large heavy-based frying pan, add the spring onions and curry powder and fry over a medium heat for 2 to 3 minutes. Add the mushrooms and continue to fry for a further minute before adding the rice. Coat the rice well in the curry mixture, pour the hot stock over the rice, stir, then cover with a tight-fitting lid and cook over a gentle heat for 30 minutes or until the rice is just cooked.

2. Remove the lid and stir in the fish, peas, tomatoes, parsley and lemon juice, heat through for 2 to 3 minutes, then season to taste with freshly ground black pepper.

3. Serve topped with the egg quarters sprinkled with a pinch of cayenne and the chopped nuts scattered over the top. Serve with a lemon wedge.

Ingredients

1 tablespoon rapeseed or vegetable oil
8 spring onions, thinly sliced
1 tablespoon medium curry powder
75g mushrooms, sliced
300g brown basmati rice
600ml reduced-sodium chicken or vegetable stock, simmering
250g smoked mackerel or kipper fillets, skinned
100g frozen peas
8 cherry tomatoes, halved
3 tablespoons chopped fresh parsley
2 teaspoons lemon juice
Freshly ground black pepper
4 medium eggs, hard boiled, peeled and quartered
Pinch of cayenne pepper
3 Brazil nuts, chopped
6 almonds, chopped

| Per serving: 735 kcals | 33g protein | 39g fat | 8g saturated fat | 68g carbs | 4g sugar | 6g fibre | 1.6g salt |

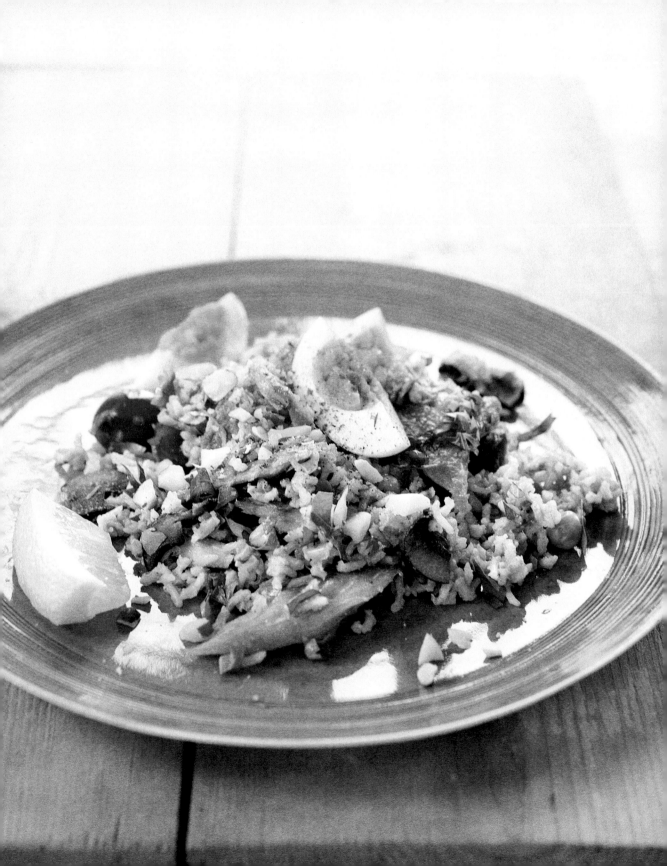

CANCER

Cancer is the diagnosis that everyone dreads. It's not the death sentence it used to be twenty or thirty years ago, but it is still a life-changing condition, even after sufferers are free of the disease. There is a genetic link in some cancers, but leading a healthy lifestyle can significantly reduce your risk.

THE SCIENCE

Cancer is the unregulated growth of any component of the body's tissues, leading to destruction of the organs or depletion of the immune and nutritional systems. The most common cancers in the UK are lung, bowel, breast and prostate, but any part of the body can be affected. Some cancers affect the tissues that normally produce hormones, such as the ovary or adrenal gland, and these can exert metabolic effects. Tumours of solid tissues can secrete by-products into the blood that affect the way we feel; for example, they might trigger the adrenal system to produce adrenaline so that we are constantly on edge.

PREVENTION

The body thrives on variety. All its physiological processes – heart rate, breathing, digestion, and so forth – require periods of activity, periods of rest, periods of stress and periods of relaxation, to keep all the tissues functioning normally. Exercise is crucial for giving a range of stimulation. A varied diet has the same effect.

However, avoidance of cancer-causing agents is also important. If tissues are constantly exposed to them they can change towards a cancerous state, where they break free from the normal regulatory processes and may go on to become a full-blown tumour. This can be caused by smoking, excess alcohol, excessive unprotected sun exposure, over-stimulation of the breast with hormones (such as HRT), or environmental irritants (such as asbestos) affecting lung tissue. Unremitting emotional stress may also be a risk factor.

IF YOU ARE DIAGNOSED WITH CANCER

It is crucial to be conscientious about good nutrition and to try to get your nutrient stores up to the maximum in preparation for treatment. Chemotherapy and surgery can be arduous, but good reserves of nutrients will help you to get through and minimize the risk of complications. Nausea, vomiting and diarrhoea are common side effects of chemotherapy. Aim to eat small portions of foods that are not rich or sickly but contain maximum nutrients. Wet foods, with sauces and gravy, are better than dry, although crackers can ease nausea. Cooking smells can increase nausea so it may be best to choose cold foods. If you get a sore mouth from chemo, or find a bitter taste left in your mouth, swishing around some pineapple juice can help. Suck ice chips to stay hydrated. And try ginger to ease nausea: drink ginger tea (see recipe on page 167), suck ginger sweets or nibble ginger biscuits.

Foods to Eat

- **Eat plenty of fresh fruits and vegetables that are high in antioxidant vitamins A, C, E and selenium,** which can neutralize harmful free radicals formed by our metabolic processes. In most cases, the best sources of vitamin C are raw rather than cooked, which is why some people recommend raw juice diets, but on the whole it's better to eat the whole fruit or veg for the fibre content. Some nutrients are easier to absorb when cooked so aim for a mix of raw and cooked.

- **Make sure your diet has enough fibre to keep your bowels working efficiently:** include pulses and whole grains in your diet at every meal.
- **Eat plenty of omega 3 fats** (olive oil, oily fish, nuts, seeds).
- **Use healthy cooking methods,** such as steaming or stir frying, as overcooking will leach the nutrients.

Foods to Avoid

- **Avoid eating a lot of red meat (no more than 500g per week) and avoid processed meats** such as sausages, bacon, ham, salami, corned beef and pies. High consumption has been implicated in a higher risk of bowel cancer.
- **Avoid transfats (aka hydrogenated fats),** found in many shop-bought cakes, biscuits and processed foods.
- **Limit your consumption of salty foods,** because there is evidence linking salt with stomach cancer.
- **Pickled, vinegary foods** have also been linked to stomach cancer.
- **Avoid charred foods,** for example meats over-cooked on a barbecue, or grilled or fried on a high heat.

Expert Tip

- **Cancer Research** (www.cancerresearchuk.org) recommendations for cancer prevention are that you stay as slim as possible without being underweight; are physically active for at least thirty minutes a day; and limit your consumption of high-calorie foods and sugary drinks.

WARNING

Consult your GP if you have any of the following: an unusual new lump on the body; blood in your stools, urine, spit or vomit; nausea and loss of appetite; a persistent cough; changes in bowel habits; unexplained distension of the abdomen; unexplained breathlessness; unexplained weight loss; or if you feel unusally tired or run down.

CASE STUDY

Peter is a sixty-two-year-old businessman, who leads a hectic life. He noticed over the course of a few months that he was getting up two or three times a night to pass urine and when he got to the loo it was taking a while to start to flow. He had also noticed a backache. After visiting his GP, he was referred for an examination of his prostate gland, an x-ray and a blood test. Unfortunately, they found he had prostate cancer, which had spread to his vertebrae, causing the back pain. Peter needed radiotherapy treatment on his vertebrae, and a combination of hormone and chemotherapy for the prostate cancer. He had to be in good nutritional condition to maximize the benefits of treatment, so attention to his diet was vital. He was advised to eat plenty of fresh fruit and veg, especially tomatoes, and he was told that reducing animal fats and dairy products, and replacing them with fish and olive oil, could help remove 'pro-cancer' substances from his diet. Some of the hormone treatment would reduce his bone density, so attention to his vitamin D and calcium intake was essential. He could take tofu or other soya products, kale or kidney beans, to help with this.

CARDIOVASCULAR DISEASE

Doctors use cardiovascular disease (CVD) as an umbrella term for a number of diseases that affect the arteries. These include peripheral vascular disease, in which arteries become narrowed in the legs and feet and sufferers experience claudication, a kind of cramp in the leg, when they are walking or climbing stairs. Narrowing of the arteries in the heart is called coronary heart disease, which can lead to angina (a kind of 'heart cramp') and/or a heart attack. There are many possible causes of heart failure, which occurs when the heart is no longer able to pump enough blood to keep the organs functioning properly. And narrowed arteries in the brain make you more prone to strokes. Altogether, cardiovascular disease is the leading cause of premature death in the UK, with one in three men and one in five women dying prematurely because of it – which seems a terrible shame, when there is so much that can be done to prevent it.

THE SCIENCE

Arteries can become narrowed by deposits of cholesterol that turn into plaques, which can bleed and clot, cutting the flow of blood; or by a blood clot that breaks off and travels from a large artery to a small one and blocks it. You are more at risk of this happening if you smoke, drink excessive amounts of alcohol, are overweight or obese, if you don't take regular exercise that raises your heart rate, if you eat a diet containing a lot of saturated fats, or if you lead a stressful lifestyle. High blood pressure, high cholesterol and diabetes all make you more likely to get CVD. It's obvious that to prevent it, you should avoid these risk factors as far as you possibly can.

If your risk of developing CVD is high, you may be prescribed medication: drugs called statins or firbrates to lower blood cholesterol; one of a number of drugs to reduce blood pressure; or an anticoagulant such as warfarin, which can reduce the risk of clotting. Some susceptible people are advised to take a low-dose aspirin daily to protect them against clotting and certain researchers in the field have even suggested that it could be beneficial for everyone over the age of fifty to take a daily 75mg aspirin. However, others point out that while your risk of heart disease can be decreased by a daily aspirin, your risk of unwanted bleeding could be increased, along with the risk of stomach ulcers. Look at your family history before deciding whether or not to take a low-dose aspirin and if you are receiving treatment for any other conditions, check with your doctor or specialist before starting.

A diet aimed at preventing cardiovascular disease would address your particular risk factors. If you have high blood pressure, you should follow the DASH diet (see page 240). If you have high cholesterol, follow the Portfolio diet (see page 244). And if you have both, a dietitian will help to devise a plan that combines the benefits of both diets for you.

Foods to Eat

- **Eat a low-fat, high-fibre diet with lots of different fruits and vegetables** to benefit your general, as well as your cardiovascular, health. Use the Mediterranean diet (lots of vegetables, whole grains, fish and olive oil, with very little red meat) as your template, unless you are already following the DASH or Portfolio diets.

- **Oily fish** – salmon (see recipe on page 231), mackerel, herring, trout, sardines – can help to stop clots forming and prevent arrythmia of the heart. Eat two or three portions a week. Include lots of avocados, nuts and seeds in your diet, and use olive or rapeseed oils for cooking and salad dressings.

- **Garlic, onions and ginger have anticoagulant properties,** so add them to stir-fries and sauces.

- **Keeping yourself well hydrated** is important.

Foods to Avoid

- **Saturated fats:** this means red meat, processed meats (such as sausages and burgers), butter, lard, cream, cheese, cakes, biscuits, pastry, and anything containing palm oil or coconut oil.

- **Keep salt intake as low as possible.** Cook from fresh to avoid the high levels of salt added to ready-prepared foods. Use 'low salt' salts and include spices and herbs to add flavour.

- **Keep alcohol consumption below the government recommended levels** of two to three units a day for women and three to four for men. However, one to two units a day for men over forty and post-menopausal women may slightly reduce the risk of heart disease.

Expert Tips

- **If you haven't exercised for years, are over forty or are obese, don't launch into a strenuous exercise programme without the supervision of a qualified instructor.** It's asking for trouble to put that kind of strain on your heart. Get your instructor to design a programme that will start gently and build up gradually. The standard advice is that you should do thirty minutes of exercise five days a week, but even a ten-minute walk is worth doing if this is all you can manage.

- **It's scary to be told you have heart disease or CVD.** Every time your heart beats a bit faster than normal, you might be worrying that you're about to have a heart attack. Read up on the subject – the British Heart Foundation website www.bhf.org.uk is a good starting point – but don't become obsessed to the point that it takes over your life. Learn relaxation techniques if you think you need to relax more.

WARNING

Around a quarter of heart attacks in people under the age of forty are related to cocaine use. You are nearly twenty-five times more likely to have one in the first hour after use, even if you are otherwise healthy. The effects of the drug are to narrow the arteries and raise the blood pressure, so it's a bit of a no-brainer. This is so prevalent now that if doctors see a young city type admitted to A&E with chest pains, they will automatically suspect cocaine could be a factor.

See also: High blood pressure, High cholesterol, Diabetes, Stroke

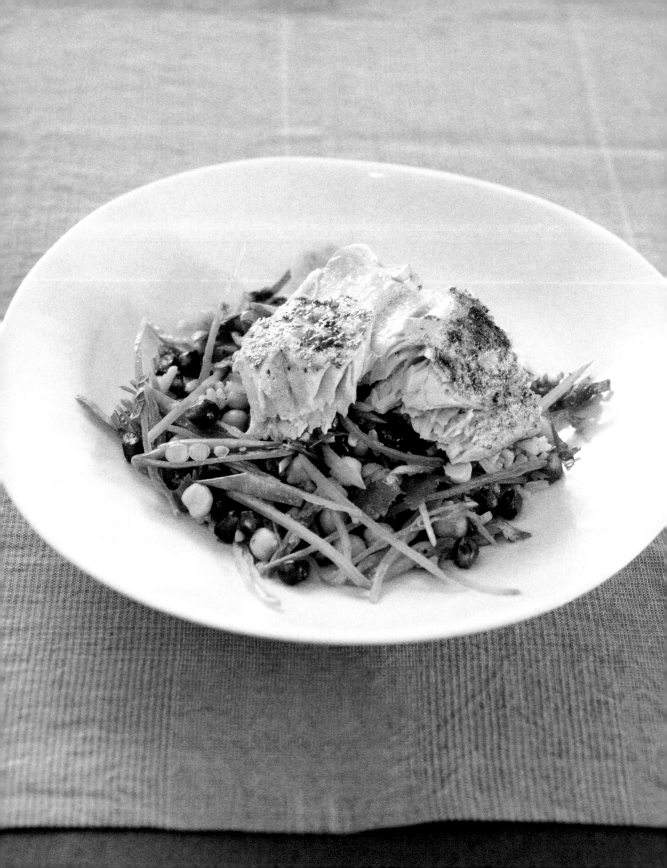

SPICY
BAKED FISH

Serves 4
Preparation time: 15 minutes
Cooking time: 30 minutes

1. Preheat oven to 200°C/180° fan/gas 6.

2. Cook the rice as per pack instructions, drain and refresh.

3. Meanwhile, prepare and combine the remaining salad ingredients in a large bowl, adding the rice once cooked, drained and refreshed. Put to one side.

4. Brush a roasting tin with a little of the oil. Wash and dry the fish, place in the roasting tin. Mix the remaining oil with the Cajun seasoning and brush liberally all over the fish. Bake uncovered for 15 minutes or until fish flakes with a fork.

5. Slice the salmon into 4 pieces and serve with spoonfuls of the salad.

Ingredients

1 tablespoon olive oil
450g salmon fillet
1 teaspoon salt-free Cajun seasoning

For the Salad

200g easy-cook wholegrain brown rice
1 x 400g tin chickpeas, rinsed and drained
100g mangetout, shredded
100g sugarsnap peas, shredded
1 x 110g pack freshly prepared pomegranate seeds
1 tablespoon olive oil
Finely grated zest and juice of 1 lime
20g mint, leaves only, roughly chopped
20g coriander, roughly chopped
Freshly ground black pepper

Per serving: 540 kcals	33g protein	2g fat	3.5g saturated fat	57g carbs	7g sugar	7g fibre	0.49g salt

DIABETES

Diabetes is caused by a failure of the blood sugar regulation mechanism so that your blood glucose levels build up, and the way you process carbohydrate, fat and protein becomes abnormal as a result. It's a serious disease because it causes all sorts of other conditions, including clogged-up arteries, damage to the kidneys, leg ulcers and gangrene, problems with eyesight and immune system malfunctions.

Symptoms can include fatigue, excessive thirst and passing urine. If you keep a jug of water by your bed and have emptied it by morning, and if you have to get up to pass water three or four times a night, it's worth getting a blood test, which your GP can arrange.

THE SCIENCE

There are two types of diabetes. In Type 1 diabetes, the beta cells in your pancreas completely stop producing insulin, the hormone used to regulate blood sugar. It is thought this could be triggered by either a virus, or possibly by your own immune system attacking the beta cells, but no one knows for sure. You no longer have sufficient insulin to deal with any sugar in your blood and if your levels rise too high you will fall into a coma and die. It is crucial that you get medical help to control your insulin levels and work out a long-term management plan. This type of diabetes typically affects younger people.

In Type 2 diabetes, your pancreas still produces insulin, but either it is not producing enough or your body is resistant to the presence of it, as if it wasn't there. Most mild cases can be controlled with diet alone or you may require oral medication. If you have a family history of Type 2 diabetes, it's imperative that you keep your weight within normal levels, eat a low-GL diet, and cut back on sugary foods that cause blood sugar swings and put pressure on the regulatory mechanism. Sometimes, women get an early warning sign during pregnancy, when they get 'gestational diabetes'. This usually goes away after the pregnancy, but it's a warning of things to come.

If you are diabetic, it's important to go for regular health checks so you can keep an eye on your blood pressure and blood cholesterol, your feet and eyesight, to try to avoid developing any of the complications of the disease. The better your control, the fewer complications you will get.

Foods to Eat

- **If you are taking insulin to control your diabetes,** you may be put on a system whereby you count your carb intake and calculate how much insulin you need to give yourself to balance your blood sugar. This gives diabetics much more freedom with their diet than they had in the past.

- **Whether you are taking insulin or not, stick to low-GL foods** to keep your blood sugar steady.

- **There is some evidence that cinnamon** can help to reduce blood sugar levels: sprinkle some on your porridge, or add it to cooked apple.

- **The flavinols in dark chocolate seemed to increase insulin sensitivity in a recent trial.** Subjects who took 100g a day found their sugar metabolism significantly improved (see recipe on page 235).

- **Magnesium, chromium, zinc and vitamin B3 all help to stabilize blood sugar.** Eat plenty of dairy products, green vegetables, whole grains, bananas, black pepper, brewer's yeast, seafood and pulses to ensure you aren't deficient in these.

- **Drink lots of water** (not squash or sugary drinks) to keep yourself hydrated.

Foods to Avoid

- **Saturated or transfat.** You're at a higher risk of CVA so avoid raising you cholestrol.

- **Excess alcohol will put pressure on your blood sugar regulation.** Never drink on an empty stomach, and if you have been drinking, always eat something low GL before going to bed to help stabilize your blood sugar.

- **Traditional products for diabetics** are full of fat and artificial sweeteners and best avoided.

Expert Tips

- **Regular cardiovascular exercise really improves insulin sensitivity.** Try to do something that makes you out of breath for thirty minutes every day.

- **If you've been diagnosed with diabetes**, regular monitoring is essential to avoid complications.

WARNING

If you are worried that you might have diabetes, get tested straight away. There are many nasty complications of the disease that can be prevented with careful management.

See also: Heart disease, High blood pressure, High cholesterol, Kidney disease

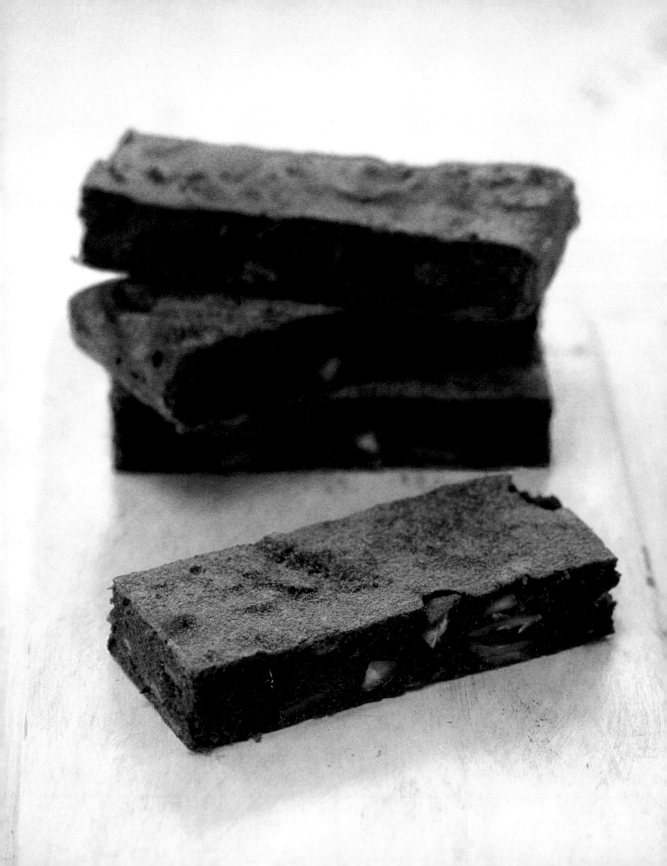

BROWNIES

Makes 15 brownies
Preparation time: 15 minutes
Cooking time: 20 minutes

Ingredients

1. Preheat oven to 180°C/160°C fan/gas 4. Lightly grease a 29 x 21cm brownie tin with a little olive oil spread. Line the tin using non-stick greaseproof paper and put to one side while you make your brownie mixture.

2. Over a medium heat combine the apple juice, dates and prunes in a small saucepan and bring to the boil. Reduce the heat to low and simmer for 2 to 3 minutes or until all the apple juice has been absorbed and the fruit has clearly softened. Using a wooden spoon, beat to form a sticky paste, set aside to cool.

3. To a large mixing bowl, add the eggs, olive oil spread, sugar, vanilla essence, drinking chocolate, cocoa and flour, and beat together using an electric whisk until just combined. Now stir in the fruit paste, dark chocolate and nuts.

4. Spoon the mixture into the prepared tin and bake for 12 to 15 minutes or until it has a crisp shell on the top and is just firm to touch – do not over-cook as the brownies will go dry. Leave to cool in the tin and divide into 15 bars. Dust with the cinnamon and serve.

100ml fresh apple juice

90g unsweetened stoned dates, chopped

90g ready-to-eat prunes, chopped

4 eggs, beaten

5 tablespoons olive oil spread

75g dark muscovado sugar

1 tablespoon vanilla essence

4 tablespoons low-cal drinking choc, e.g. Options/Cadbury Highlights

2 tablespoons cocoa powder

175g plain flour

100g dark chocolate (minimum 70 per cent cocoa), broken into small pieces

30g pistachios, roughly chopped

30g flaked almonds

1 teaspoon ground cinnamon

| Per serving: 206 kcals | 5g protein | 11g fat | 3g saturated fat | 24g carbs | 14g sugar | 2g fibre | 0.26g salt |

EPILEPSY

Epileptic seizures occur when there is an uncontrolled frenzy of electrical activity in the brain. Sometimes they can be quite mild, affecting the areas of the brain that control perception, such as smell. In a full-blown or generalized seizure, the sufferer loses consciousness and collapses, may shake uncontrollably, dribble and be incontinent. In theory, anyone can have a seizure: sleep deprivation and alcohol can induce one in people who are not otherwise epileptic. But those with epilepsy suffer from them on a regular basis, and in these cases anti-epilepsy medication is usually prescribed and prevents seizures in around seventy per cent of sufferers.

THE SCIENCE

There are different causes of epilepsy. Some people have a localized trigger area in the brain where seizures start. An abnormal group of cells that they were born with may be responsible. Sometimes epilepsy can follow trauma to the brain, such as after an accident, a stroke or an infection like meningitis. It can also be caused by certain metabolic conditions in which glucose cannot get into the brain.

There can be triggers that stimulate the brain in such a way as to set off a seizure. For example, most people are aware that flashing lights at a certain frequency can trigger one type of epilepsy, leading to a seizure. Television programmes issue warnings about flashing lights so that sufferers can avoid them.

People with epilepsy usually get some kind of warning signs that a seizure is imminent, known as a 'prodrome'. Typically this might be a visual aura and a sense that all is not well. If sufferers learn to recognize the signs, they can get themselves into a safe position in a safe place and summon help before it progresses.

The first line of treatment for epilepsy is anti-epileptic medication, but this doesn't work for around a quarter of children. Alternative treatment options could include surgery, vagus nerve stimulation treatment or a ketogenic diet. The diet is considered for children whose seizures fail to respond to treatment with at least two anti-epileptic medications. The diet is also used for children with certain metabolic disorders (Glucose transporter 1 deficiency and Pyruvate Dehydrogenase deficiency) or patients who have intolerable side effects from anti-epileptic medication. It is high in fat with adequate protein and low carbs to help recreate the metabolic changes that occur when the body is fasting. It's not fully understood why it reduces seizures but it can be very effective. There is some research that is looking at the effect of the diet in adults with medication-resistant epilepsy as well.

But don't try to put yourself on it: the ketogenic diet should only ever be followed under the supervision of a qualified medical specialist. Portions are carefully calorie-controlled to stop you gaining too much weight. It is a very difficult diet to follow because all foods must be weighed and the exact quantities eaten that the dietitian recommends. It is not safe to start following this diet without help. (You'll find more information about it on the Great Ormond Street Hospital website www.gosh.nhs.uk.)

Foods to Eat

- **Ordinarily, in most individuals with epilepsy, there are no particular foods that affect the occurrence of seizures.** However, a ketogenic diet might be recommended as a treatment. Some people use a modified Atkins-style diet or a low-GL diet instead, as they are easier to follow (the recipe on page 238 is a high-fat, low-carb meal). Ask your dietitian what would be best in your case.

Foods to Avoid

- **If you think certain foods (or the smell of certain foods) might trigger attacks, start keeping a detailed diary of foods eaten, external circumstances, and when seizures occur.** If you suspect a particular food, omit it from your diet for four weeks to see if the frequency of seizures lessens then reintroduce it again and monitor the effects.

Expert Tips

- **You may need other people to describe what happens to you during a seizure.** Even if you don't collapse on the floor, you might not be aware of what's going on.
- **Some children have 'absence seizures',** and these are often picked up when they appear inattentive in class. They will be quiet and seem to be daydreaming, rather than being rowdy and disruptive.
- **If you suffer from epileptic seizures, you may be advised to wear a MedicAlert bracelet** so that you can be given appropriate help if you collapse somewhere.

- **You may be best advised to avoid dangerous situations,** such as standing on the edge of cliffs!
- **If you are a driver and are diagnosed as epileptic,** you can only drive once you have been completely seizure-free for twelve months, or if you experience sleep seizures only, if you have been seizure-free for three years.
- **If you haven't had a seizure for many years and are still taking medication,** it may be worth seeing a neurologist to review whether you still need it.

CASE STUDY

At the age of seven, Jessica was having epileptic seizures once or twice a day, despite the fact that she was taking two different kinds of medication to try and control it. Her specialist brought in a dietitian, who helped to put her on a ketogenic diet. It's a difficult diet to get used to, but fortunately Jessica's mother was a good cook and she was able to develop some different recipes that Jessica enjoyed eating. Within a few months, the incidence of seizures was down to just one a week. Jessica needs to have her blood tested regularly to make sure she is not suffering any adverse effects, but it seems to have been a successful strategy for the management of her epilepsy.

WARNING

If you black out, even if just for a few seconds, you must see a doctor.

CREAMY CHICKEN AND TARRAGON

Serves 4
Preparation time: 5 minutes
Cooking time: 45 minutes

Ingredients

1. Heat the butter and oil in a small casserole dish or saucepan. When the butter starts to foam, add the chicken thighs, cook skin side down for 5 minutes over a medium to high heat, then turn over and cook for a further 5 minutes or until golden on both sides. Season with freshly ground black pepper, add the mushrooms and garlic to the pan and fry for 5 minutes more.

2. Pour the stock into the pan, bring to the boil and then reduce the heat to a gentle simmer, cook for 30 minutes, stirring once after 15 minutes. Once the chicken thighs are cooked through, pour in the cream and add the tarragon, and continue to simmer for 2 to 3 minutes.

3. Serve with steamed curly kale or cauliflower.

25g unsalted butter
1½ tablespoons olive oil
8 chicken thighs, skin on and bone in
Freshly ground black pepper
150g chestnut mushrooms, halved, or quartered if large
2 cloves garlic, peeled and crushed
500ml chicken stock
100ml double cream
2 tablespoons chopped tarragon leaves

To Serve

Steamed cauliflower or curly kale

Per serving: 466 kcals | 47g protein | 31g fat | 15g saturated fat | 1g carbs | 0.5g sugar | 0.8g fibre | 0.6g salt

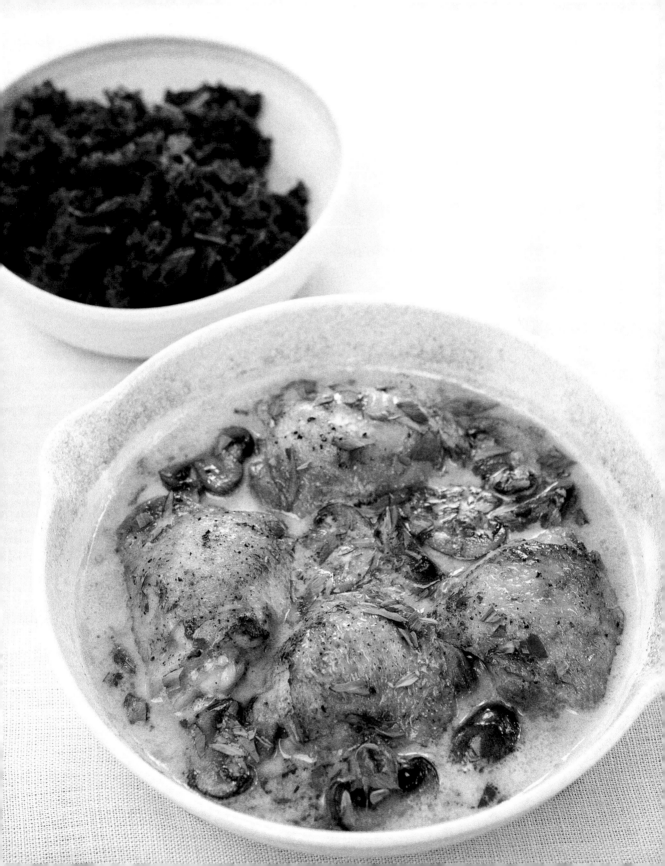

HIGH BLOOD PRESSURE

In ninety per cent of cases, there is no obvious cause for high blood pressure. Doctors call this 'essential hypertension'. It goes up in most of us as we age, but unless there are other health conditions present, it shouldn't go above 140 over 90. That's a guide. If you are diabetic or have kidney disease, you should aim even lower than this: 120 over 80 is the ideal.

You may not know you have high blood pressure because it doesn't cause any symptoms, but it puts you at greatly increased risk of heart attack, kidney disease or stroke. There are some health problems we can't do much about – they're just down to genetics and bad luck – but taking our blood pressure in hand is something we can all do if we want to lead a longer, healthier life.

THE SCIENCE

Men whose waist measurement is over 102cm and women with a waist over 88cm are more at risk of high blood pressure. For Asians, it's less than this: 90cm for men and 80cm for women. So, the first thing you can do to prevent (or reduce) high blood pressure is to get your weight down to within the healthy range for your height (see the BMI chart on page 59).

Regular exercise will reduce blood pressure and you should aim to do thirty minutes minimum a day of cardiovascular exercise – the kind that makes you out of breath and raises your heart rate. Stress is also bad for blood pressure, so it's important to find ways of dealing with any stress in your life and scheduling in regular periods of relaxation.

Smoking is just about the worst thing you can do if you have high blood pressure, and drinking excessive quantities of alcohol is right behind it.

There's loads of nutritional advice that can help you to keep your blood pressure healthy, and something called the DASH diet has been very successful in helping people to lower their blood pressure. The acronym stands for Dietary Approaches to Stop Hypertension, and the first principle is that you cut right back on the amount of salt you take. Salt is a huge villain in the fight to control blood pressure. If the whole population of the UK cut down to just 3g of salt a day, we could prevent 30,000 deaths a year. For more on this, see the website www.actiononsalt.org.uk, where you will find loads of useful advice and interesting facts.

On the DASH diet, you eat seven to eight small portions of whole grains a day, four to five portions of fruits and four to five of vegetables, two to three low-fat dairy portions, two portions (or fewer) of lean meat, fish or poultry, four to five portions a week of nuts, seeds and legumes, and a very limited amount of fat and sugar. For more information, go to www.dashdiet.org. It's a very healthy diet, but check with your doctor before starting it, just in case there are any special circumstances that would make it unsuitable.

Foods to Eat

- **Eat a low-fat, high-fibre diet,** with plenty of antioxidant-containing fruits and vegetables (see recipe on page 243).
- **Potassium helps to flush excess sodium** (salt) from your body, so eat lots of potatoes, bananas, oranges and apricots. Calcium and magnesium are also important elements of the DASH diet due to their regulating effects on blood pressure.
- **High blood pressure can be linked to vitamin D deficiency,** so get plenty of oily fish and sunshine. Oily fish is also an anticoagulant, and helps to prevent arrhythmia of the heart.
- **In studies, eating soya protein lowered the blood pressure** of participants, but note that men and pre-menopausal women shouldn't eat too much soya. Just have some as part of a balanced, varied diet.
- **Eating 45g of dark chocolate containing eighty-five per cent cocoa** solids per day helped reduce high blood pressure in a number of different trials.
- **Garlic powder capsules** have been shown to reduce blood pressure, and ginger can also have beneficial effects.

Foods to Avoid

- **Cutting back on salt** has been found in study after study to lower blood pressure and reduce the risk of cardiovascular disease and stroke. Watch out for products with hidden salt, such as tinned soups, processed foods and fast foods. Read food labels.

- **Grapefruit and grapefruit juice should be avoided** when you are on certain kinds of blood pressure medication called calcium channel blockers. Check with your doctor.
- **Alcohol raises blood pressure,** so cut right down to no more than one alcoholic drink a day.

Expert Tip

When trying to reduce your blood pressure, it's a good idea to keep a food diary to increase your awareness of what you're eating. It's easy to pop leftovers in your mouth without thinking, but it will focus the mind when you know you have to write every single item down.

CASE STUDY

At a routine eye test, Shirley was told that she had some changes in her eyes that might be due to high blood pressure. She didn't have any symptoms, but she checked it using a machine in a pharmacy and it read 165 over 98 – far too high. She went to her GP, and he organized some further tests and prescribed medication. Shirley took up brisk walking every day and reduced the salt in her diet. These combined measures brought her blood pressure down and in turn reduced her risk of heart disease and stroke.

WARNING

High blood pressure is a silent killer, so get yours checked once a year.

See also: Cardiovascular disease, Stroke

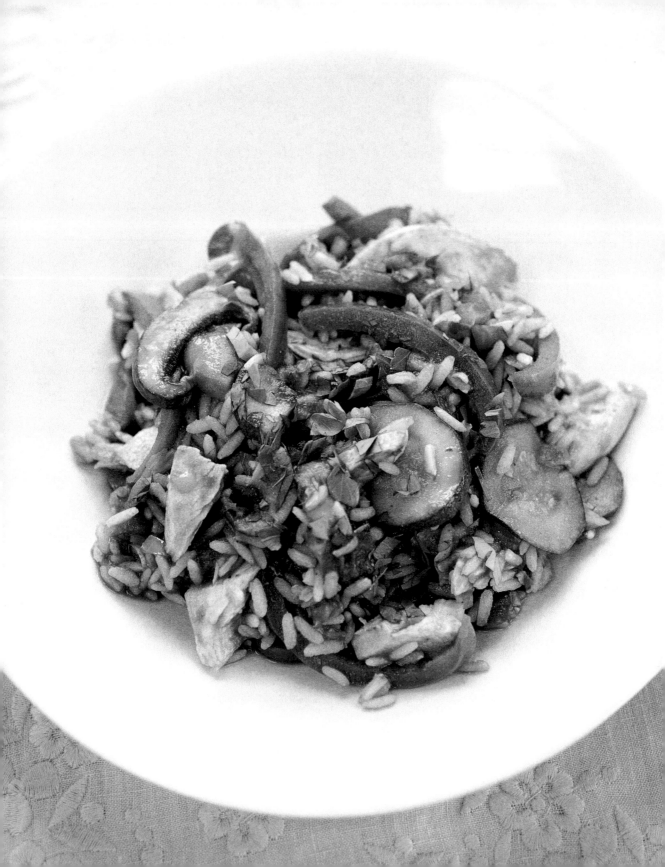

CHICKEN AND SPANISH RICE

Serves 4
Preparation time: 5 minutes
Cooking time: 25 minutes

1. Cook the rice as per pack instructions.

2. Cook the onions in the oil for 5 minutes over a medium heat, add the garlic, pepper, mushrooms and courgette and cook for a further 5 minutes.

3. Add the tinned tomatoes, puree and chilli to the pan and simmer for 5 minutes, season to taste with freshly ground black pepper.

4. Drain the rice and add to the pan with the vegetables, along with the chicken and parsley. Heat through for 5 minutes and serve.

Ingredients

400g easy-cook wholegrain rice

2 onions, finely chopped

2 teaspoons rapeseed or olive oil

2 cloves garlic, crushed

1 green pepper, deseeded and sliced

4 chestnut mushrooms, chopped

½ courgette, thinly sliced

1 x 400g tin chopped tomatoes

2 tablespoons tomato puree

1–2 teaspoons medium chilli powder

Freshly ground black pepper

325g cooked chicken, chopped into bite-sized pieces

1 teaspoon flat leaf parsley, finely chopped

| Per serving: 537 kcals | 34g protein | 8g fat | 2g saturated fat | 89g carbs | 8g sugar | 5g fibre | 0.3g salt |

HIGH CHOLESTEROL

Cholesterol has got a bad name of late but, in fact, we need a certain amount of it for essential body processes, such as the manufacture of hormones and the insulation of nerve endings. Most of the cholesterol we need is made in the liver, from the fatty foods we eat, but the problem is that high levels in the blood can clog up our arteries with fatty plaque deposits and make us more likely to have a heart attack or stroke.

THE SCIENCE

Cholesterol is transported in the blood in low-density lipoproteins (LDL) and high-density lipoproteins (HDL), and it's the LDL variety that is bad news (L = lousy!). When we eat fatty foods, the fat is transported in the blood in a form called triglycerides, and high levels of these will also increase the likelihood of heart problems. Cholesterol levels can only be confirmed by a blood test. Total cholesterol of under 5 mmol/litre is the recommended level, but in the UK, an alarming two out of three adults have higher levels than this.

You may not find out that you have a problem until you start experiencing symptoms of clogged-up arteries, or atherosclerosis. These include chest pain (angina), leg pain when exercising, blood clots and ruptured blood vessels, or a mini-stroke, stroke or heart attack.

High cholesterol levels can be a genetic trend, and if you have inherited it you may have a white ring around the iris in your eye, known as an arcus, or fatty patches on the skin around the eyes called xanthalasma. Lifestyle is all-important in keeping cholesterol levels at a healthy level, though. A diet containing a lot of saturated fat will increase your risk, as will not getting enough exercise, being overweight and drinking excessive amounts of alcohol. The older you are, the more your risk of high cholesterol levels, and people of Indian, Pakistani, Bangladeshi and Sri Lankan descent appear to have a predisposition to higher levels.

Prevention is much easier than cure. If you have a close relative who has suffered from a cholesterol-related condition, you should take special care. If you are found to have high levels, you may be prescribed medication like statins, or be told to take a daily dose of soluble aspirin, but any medication should be taken in combination with lifestyle modifications. A new diet, known as the Portfolio Diet, has been achieving extraordinary results, reducing harmful cholesterol levels by as much as twenty-five per cent. You can download information about the diet from www.heartuk.org.uk or ask your doctor, but some of the general principles are listed below. Don't self-prescribe it; check with your GP before starting in case there are any reasons why it's not suitable for you.

- **Eat a diet that's high in fibre** and rich in fruit and vegetables (see recipe on page 246).
- **If you have high cholesterol,** choose foods with 2–3g of plant stanols and sterols a day, such as a fortified mini yoghurt drink or spreads that actively block cholesterol absorption from the gut. They can achieve reductions of bad LDL cholesterol by ten to fifteen per cent.
- **Eat 30g (about 23) almonds a day.** All nuts are good, but almonds are best for their high vitamin E content, and also because they seem to reduce the levels of certain proteins used in the manufacture of LDL cholesterol.
- **Eat 20g of soluble fibre a day.** This is found in oats, oatmeal, barley, beans, pulses and apples. You would need two good portions so, for example, porridge for breakfast and pulses with your main meal. The fibre can trap some of the cholesterol in our digestive system and get rid of it before it's absorbed.
- **Eat 50g of soya protein a day:** a pint of soya milk provides about 20g, and you could also eat soya yoghurts, soya beans, and add soya mince or tofu to casseroles and stir-fries.

- **Cut right back on saturated fat.** If you want to eat red meat, cut off all visible fat, and avoid fatty meat products such as sausages and burgers.
- **Avoid butter, ghee, lard and dripping**, and opt for healthy spreads and oils.
- **Avoid full-fat dairy products,** choosing lower-fat options such as skimmed milk and no-fat yoghurt.
- **Avoid cakes,** biscuits, chocolate, pies and pastries.
- **Avoid pre-packaged meals and snacks** with a high salt content, and add as little salt as you can to your food.

- **Get thirty minutes of vigorous exercise** that makes you out of breath, five times a week.
- **Keep your weight down** at a healthy level.
- **If you have high cholesterol and you smoke**, be aware that you are basically sitting on a ticking time bomb.
- **Drinking too much alcohol** can increase your LDL and triglyceride levels.

WARNING

The links between high cholesterol and heart disease and stroke are well established. If you have a relative with cardiovascular disease, or if you have been diagnosed with high cholesterol, it's time to make some serious lifestyle changes.

See also: Cardiovascular disease; High blood pressure; Obesity and being overweight; Stroke

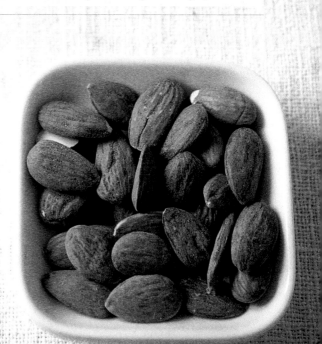

LUCY'S HEALTHY SHEPHERD'S PIE

Serves 4

Preparation time: 15 minutes

Cooking time: 1 hour

1. Preheat oven to 200°C/180° fan/gas 6.

2. Cook the sweet potatoes and squash in a steamer for 25 minutes or until tender. Mash with the olive oil spread and season with freshly ground black pepper. Put to one side.

3. Meanwhile, heat the oil in a large saucepan or casserole dish and sweat the onion over a medium to low heat, covered, for 10 minutes or until soft and translucent but not browned. Add the garlic, mushrooms and carrot and cook uncovered for 6 to 7 minutes.

4. Add the soya mince, chopped tomatoes, puree and chilli to the pan and bring to a gentle simmer for 10 minutes.

5. Add the lentils and peas to the pan and heat through, season to taste with salt and freshly ground black pepper. Spoon the mixture into a large ovenproof dish, top with the sweet potato and squash mash and scatter over the flaked almonds. Bake in the oven for 20 minutes or until the top is golden and it is piping hot throughout.

Ingredients

650g sweet potatoes, peeled and roughly chopped

300g butternut squash, peeled, deseeded and roughly chopped

20g olive-based spread

Freshly ground black pepper

1 tablespoon olive or rapeseed oil

1 onion, finely chopped

2 cloves garlic, crushed

4 chestnut mushrooms, roughly chopped

1 carrot, peeled and diced

300g frozen soya mince (or rehydrate 100g dried soya mince)

2 x 400g tins chopped tomatoes

1 tablespoon tomato puree

1–2 teaspoons chilli flakes or hot chilli powder

1 x 390g tin green lentils

150g frozen peas

Salt and freshly ground black pepper

30g flaked almonds

| Per serving: 379 kcals | 23g protein | 10g fat | 2g saturated fat | 53g carbs | 20g sugar | 13g fibre | 3.2g salt |

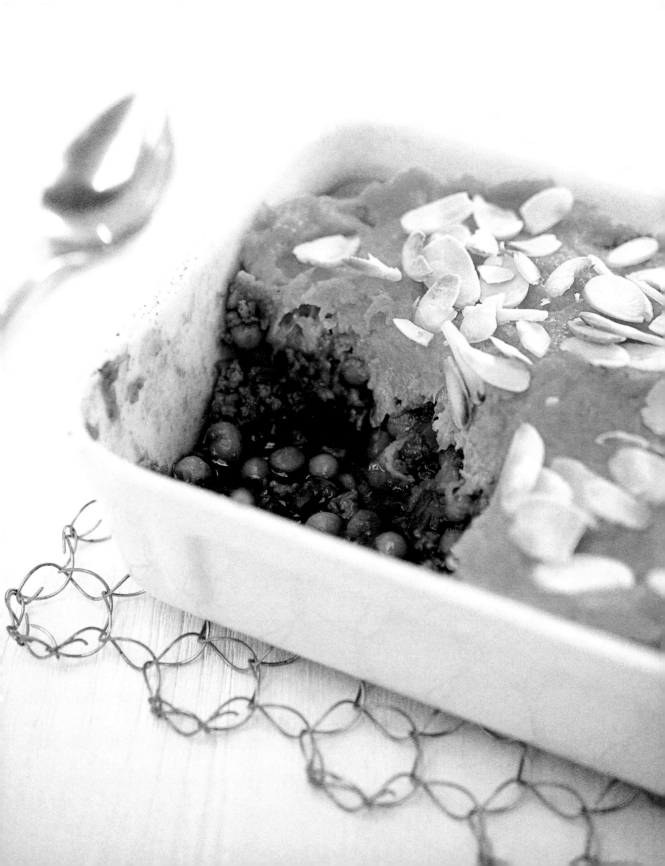

HIV

Most people are now aware that you catch human immunodeficiency virus (HIV) through contact with the body fluids (blood, semen and vaginal secretions) of someone who is already infected. The most common ways this happens are via unprotected sex or when drug users share needles. It's a devastating diagnosis for anyone to receive but it's no longer the automatic death sentence that it was when it was first detected back in the 1980s. Instead, it's often a long-term condition that requires careful management. If you hadn't particularly looked after your own health before getting this diagnosis, now is the time to start.

THE SCIENCE

The HIV virus disables the mechanisms by which your body would normally fight infection, making you susceptible to all kinds of bizarre conditions that you would never normally get if your immune system wasn't impaired. It is diagnosed by a blood test, but it can take up to six weeks after you've been exposed to the virus before the test comes up positive, so if you've had a 'risky' encounter, repeat the test two months later. After a positive diagnosis, you will be put on a drug regime, usually involving a combination of different drugs. Thereafter, you will have regular blood tests to check your CD4 count – a marker for the white blood cells that help you to fight infection – and your viral load – how much of the virus you have in your blood stream at the time.

If your CD4 counts are below 500, you may be given a treatment called HAART – standing for Highly Active Anti-Retroviral Therapy – in which three or four drugs are used in combination. Some of the side effects of HAART can cause malabsorption of nutrients in the gut, so it's important to get as wide a range of antioxidants and phytonutrients as possible. You can also be susceptible to a condition called HIV-related lipodystrophy in which your body fats are redistributed, and this can make you prone to fat build-up in the arteries, so you should follow all the usual advice for heart health: a Mediterranean diet, plenty of omega 3 fatty acids and a low intake of saturated fats.

It's crucial that you live as healthy a life as possible after diagnosis to stop your condition deteriorating, which could make you prone to opportunistic infection. People with HIV tend to burn more calories than others, and it can be a struggle to keep their weight up at healthy levels. Eating little and often will help. If you didn't cook for yourself before, buy a cookbook and get started, to enable you to eat foods containing fresh, natural ingredients, without preservatives and artificial additives, on a daily basis.

Foods to Eat

- **A Mediterranean diet** with plenty of oily fish, whole grains, nuts and seeds, fruits and vegetables. Omega 3 fish oil can help to reduce weight loss and improve immune function.

- **Eat loads of multi-coloured fruits and vegetables** – at least five or six different ones per day, more if you can manage it. Vitamin E and selenium can increase the production of antibodies: get selenium from Brazil nuts, and E from avocado, broccoli, whole grains and eggs.

- **Follow the Eatwell Plate** (see page 10), with wholegrain carbs, lean protein, vegetables, dairy and a little fat at every meal.

Foods to Avoid

- **Keep saturated fat intake low;** HAART medications can raise cholesterol levels and put sufferers at risk of heart disease.

- **Garlic supplements can interact with some HIV drugs** and reduce their effectiveness. A bit of garlic in food won't be a problem, but avoid taking large quantities in a supplement.

- **Alcohol interacts with some HAART drugs.** Check with your specialist about whether this is the case with the ones you are taking.

Expert Tips

- **Get the flu vaccine every autumn,** and you will also be offered a five-yearly vaccine against pneumococcal pneumonia, a serious chest infection.

- **Take care when handling** cat litter or animal droppings to avoid picking up the toxoplasmosis virus. Wear rubber gloves.

- **Wash your hands after going to the toilet,** travelling on public transport and before and after preparing food, to protect you from infections.

- **Getting regular exercise and not smoking** are no-brainers for anyone with HIV.

CASE STUDY

Paul was diagnosed with HIV after receiving an emergency blood transfusion while travelling abroad in a remote location some years ago. He was a smoker and quite hyperactive; he always ate on the run – which usually meant fast food and the odd smoothie. His HIV was well controlled with multiple medication but he did start to lose weight and had to boost his calorie intake. He quit smoking, took up yoga (which, initially, he hated) with a friend who already went and generally improved the overall quality of his diet. For these reasons alone, he felt a lot better in himself and actually found he took more time to enjoy life. Like reformed smokers who can't be around cigarette smoke, once he learned his way around the kitchen, Paul couldn't stand the ready meals he used to live off.

WARNING

It can be natural to feel isolated and get depressed after an HIV diagnosis, but you are not alone. It is thought that there are over 100,000 people with HIV in the UK, although at least a quarter of them may not be aware they have it. The Terrence Higgins Trust is your first stop for local counselling and support groups: www.tht.org.uk/howwecanhelpyou.

See also: Cardiovascular disease, High cholesterol

KIDNEY PROBLEMS

The kidneys are not just for producing urine; they have many different roles in our health. They play an important part in the control of calcium and phosphate levels and convert vitamin D into its active form; they have a key role in controlling blood pressure; they release a hormone that stimulates the bone marrow to produce red blood cells; and they remove waste products from the blood for excretion – among other functions. The most common things that go wrong with our kidneys are kidney stones and other kidney diseases.

KIDNEY STONES

When kidney stones pass down the urinary tract, they can cause excruciating pain that's like nothing you've ever experienced before. If they're small enough to excrete, you may be able to see them in the toilet bowl, but larger ones may require surgical removal. The commonest kinds of kidney stones (around eighty per cent) are calcium oxalates formed from excess calcium in the blood. A less common kind are struvite stones, which can form in response to urinary infections, and they grow big quite quickly. You can also get uric acid stones, which are linked to gout and are a by-product of a high-protein diet and linked to insulin resistance. The best way to protect yourself from kidney stones is to drink plenty of water, so that you are producing at least two litres of urine a day. In hot weather or during exercise, you may need to drink three or four litres of water a day to achieve this. Keep your urine from being too concentrated before your kidneys have a chance to form stones and you'll spare yourself that horrible pain! Kidney stones can also lead to complications such as kidney disease in some circumstances.

KIDNEY DISEASE

Chronic kidney disease is commonly related to high blood pressure, high cholesterol, and/or diabetes. High blood pressure damages the fine tubes within the kidney where all the magic occurs, and damage to the kidneys causes even higher blood pressure, so it's all part of a vicious circle. With kidney disease, your calcium metabolism breaks down and you're more at risk of osteoporosis. Your bone marrow can't produce enough red blood cells so you may get a form of anaemia. Diabetics are more likely to have high cholesterol, which damages the kidneys and leads to high blood pressure. All of these conditions are interlinked, and that's why early diagnosis of kidney disease is key.

A microalbuminuria test can pick up early kidney damage by detecting any proteins leaking into the urine. If you have high blood pressure or diabetes you should get this test annually. Once you are diagnosed with kidney disease, it will be even more crucial to take steps to reduce your blood pressure and cholesterol. You may need to take supplements to relieve anaemia and prevent osteoporosis. Don't self-prescribe, though. At this stage, it is important to follow the recommendations of a fully qualified dietitian, because prescription will depend on your ability to filter out potassium and phosphates – something none of us can work out for ourselves.

To prevent kidney disease, you should avoid smoking, which damages the blood vessels inside the kidney, and maintain your weight at a healthy level. Take on board all the advice for reducing high blood pressure and high cholesterol and try to keep yours within the normal range to protect your kidneys.

Foods to Eat

- **The DASH diet,** designed to lower blood pressure (see page 240), is also good for prevention of kidney stones. It is high in fruits, vegetables and legumes, low in sodium, red meat and sugary drinks. Vegetarians have a lower risk of kidney stones.
- **Probiotics containing** *oxalobacter formigenes* have been shown to increase the excretion of oxalates, so are worth trying for if you have kidnet stones.
- **Drink some cranberry juice** every day. Use the recipe on page 181 rather than shop-bought ones, which will probably contain artificial sweeteners.
- **Drink loads of plain water** every day.

Foods to Avoid

- **You should limit the amount of animal protein you eat** (meat, chicken, eggs and cheese). Official recommendations are that we eat less than 52g of protein a day, which is equivalent to around two chicken breasts.
- **Limit dietary sources of oxalate,** such as spinach, rhubarb, blueberries, beans, beets, celery, grapes, chocolate and wheat bran, which can contribute to the formation of calcium oxalate stones.
- **Calcium supplements are best avoided,** unless prescribed by your specialist.
- **Salt puts a strain on the kidneys,** so stop adding it to your food and avoid buying processed, packaged foods that are almost certain to contain it.

Expert Tips

- **The received wisdom** used to be that you should cut down on calcium if you have kidney problems – but don't self-diagnose and put yourself on a low-calcium diet, because it could upset the balance of all the other minerals in the body.
- **Get professional advice from a dietitian** if you are worried about your kidneys.

CASE STUDY

Amit's older brother had had a heart attack. While he had been a smoker and Amit wasn't, he didn't want to end up the same way so he went to see his GP. Following tests, his GP told him that he had early diabetes and high blood pressure. A urine sample showed that he had some early kidney damage as a result of these problems. Amit was surprised, because he hadn't experienced any symptoms at all. Fortunately, it was early enough to treat the blood pressure and diabetes. He switched to a healthy DASH diet, lost some weight and started an exercise regime, which improved his diabetes considerably. Now he sees his GP every three months to monitor his blood pressure and diabetes.

See also: High blood pressure, High cholesterol, Anaemia, Osteoporosis, Gout, Cystitis

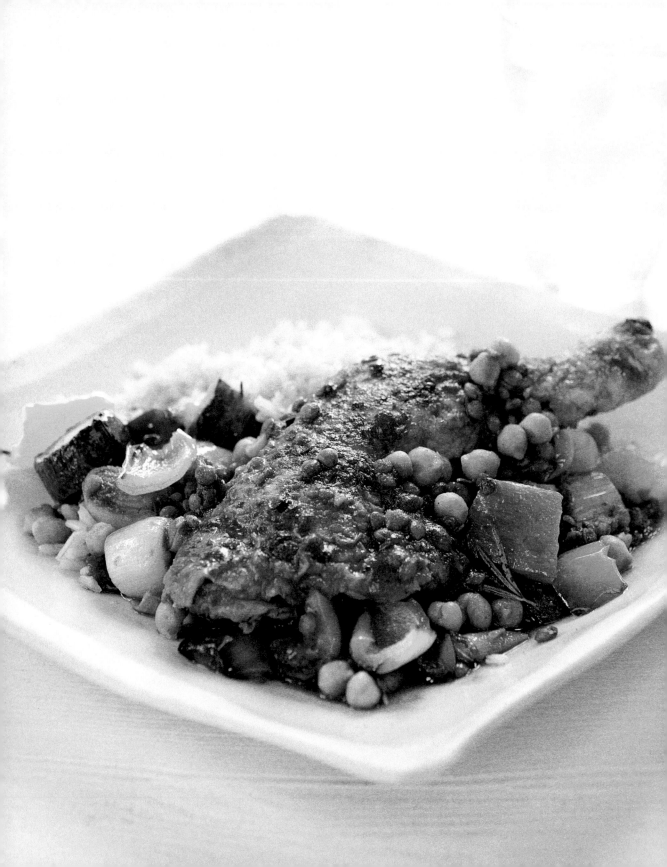

CHICKEN AND PULSE STEW

Serves 4
Preparation time: 15 minutes
Cooking time: 1 hour 20 minutes

1. Preheat the oven to 180°C/160°C fan/gas 4.

2. For the roasted vegetables, scatter all of the vegetables and rosemary in a single layer on to a large roasting tray, drizzle over the oil and toss through your fingers to coat in the oil, cook in the oven for 40 minutes or until tender and golden, turning them over half-way though.

3. For the stew, heat the oil in a large casserole, fry the chicken pieces for 10 to 12 minutes over a medium to high heat or until golden on all sides, remove from the pan using tongs, set aside and season with salt and pepper. Reduce the heat to medium and tip the leeks and garlic into the same pan and fry for 2 to 3 minutes, stirring frequently.

4. Add the remaining ingredients, stir well to combine, return the browned chicken and bring to a gentle simmer, put the lid on and place in the oven for 1 hour or until the chicken is cooked through and the stew has thickened.

5. Remove the stew from the oven and add the roasted vegetables, season to taste with salt and freshly ground black pepper. Serve with rice cooked as per pack instructions.

Ingredients

For the Roast Vegetables

1 courgette, sliced into 2.5cm thick rounds
100g butternut squash, peeled and chopped into 2.5cm pieces
1 red or yellow pepper, deseeded and sliced into chunky pieces
2 cloves garlic, peeled and bruised
3 stalks rosemary, bruised
2 tablespoons olive oil or rapeseed oil

For the Stew

1 tablespoon olive oil or rapeseed oil
1 x 2½–3 lb (1.15–1.35 kg) chicken, quartered
4 large chicken leg portions
Salt and freshly ground black pepper
3 leeks, sliced into 1-cm rounds
2 cloves garlic, peeled and crushed
1 x 400g tin chopped tomatoes
568ml salt-free fresh chicken stock
1 bay leaf
1 x 400g tin chickpeas, drained and rinsed
1 x 125g tin lentils, drained

To Serve

Brown or long grain rice

Per serving: 495 kcals | 55g protein | 20g fat | 3g saturated fat | 28g carbs | 10g sugar | 5.5g fibre | 1.1g salt

MULTIPLE SCLEROSIS

Multiple sclerosis is often in the news, as researchers battle to understand why relatively young people (normally between the ages of twenty and forty at first diagnosis) are succumbing to this extremely debilitating neurological condition in which nerves no longer transmit messages effectively from the brain to the body, causing muscle weakness, blurred vision, and difficulties with balance. There are different types of MS: relapsing-remitting, in which episodes of weakness are following by periods of remission; and progressive, in which symptoms get gradually worse over time. In the worst cases, sufferers can end up wheelchair-bound, with little muscle function left.

THE SCIENCE

No one knows why MS strikes. It has been noted that it is much less common in countries close to the equator, so there's a theory that it could be connected with a vitamin D deficiency due to lack of sun exposure in childhood. It's twice as common in women as in men and you're more likely to be diagnosed with it if there's a family history. White people are more at risk than Asians or Africans.

What happens is that the myelin sheaths around nerves, which allow them to conduct electricity and function properly, begin to deteriorate. Messages from the brain to the muscles become scrambled and slow, and gradually stop getting through at all. Diagnosis is confirmed by an MRI scan and a lumbar puncture.

In terms of prevention, since scientists don't really know the cause, all you can do is eat a varied healthy diet and maintain a healthy weight to keep your immune system in good shape. If you are diagnosed with MS, the best advice is to read as much as you can about it, join support groups and see if you can identify any triggers that bring on episodes. You may be prescribed drugs to help slow the progress of the disease and you should have access to a team of physiotherapists, speech therapists and occupational therapists, as and when you need them.

It is a life-long condition, but try not to be pessimistic. It's an area into which a lot of research funding is being poured at the moment, and while you are waiting for them to find the cure, there is a lot you can do to help yourself.

Foods to Eat

- **Alpha-linoleic acid is the big news for people with relapsing-remitting MS.** You'll find it in vegetable oils, such as corn, rapeseed, peanut, sesame, soya, sunflower, walnut and wheatgerm. It's recommended that MS sufferers get five portions of these a day, of one and a half teaspoons per portion. You may also get it from three teaspoons of polyunsaturated spreads such as sunflower or soya. The combined results of a number of double-blind studies concluded that this will reduce the severity and the duration of relapses, particularly if sufferers start taking the oils before they are severely disabled by their MS.

- **Eating 10 to 15g of walnuts,** Brazil nuts, sesame, sunflower, pumpkin or poppy seeds, or 20 to 30g of peanuts, peanut butter or almonds per day, two and a half teaspoons of full-fat mayonnaise and 35g of taramasalata can also provide the correct amount of alpha-linoleic acid.

- **You should eat oily fish two to three times a week.** Combined with increased alpha-linoleic acid, trials showed a decreased duration, frequency and severity of relapses in sufferers (see recipe on page 256).

- **Eat plenty of foods containing vitamin D:** oily fish and fortified spreads will help, but eggs, cream and cheese are also good. If you are housebound and can't get out into the sunshine, you should take a vitamin D preparation to prevent deficiency.

Foods to Avoid

- **Some MS patients try excluding foods** such as wheat, dairy and soya to see if their symptoms improve. Any evidence of this is purely anecdotal but by all means try it. Ifyou do, be careful your diet remains nutritionally balanced.

Expert Tips

- **Doing exercise to increase muscle strength** may help to retain control of them.

- **Do join support groups such as the Multiple Sclerosis Society (www.mssociety.org.uk)** and take advantage of the wisdom of other members who may have been living with the condition for longer than you.

WARNING

Get the flu jab every autumn, and a vaccination against pneumoccal pneumonia as advised by your doctor. Your immune system might not be strong enough to fight off these infections. Discuss any dietary changes you want to make with your GP or specialist before starting, just in case there are any contraindications in your case.

SMOKED MACKEREL SALAD WITH BEETROOT, SPINACH AND AVOCADO

Serves 4
Preparation time: 15 minutes
Cooking time: 5 minutes

1. Gently toast the pumpkin seeds in a small frying pan over a medium heat for 2 to 3 minutes, and tip on to kitchen paper to cool.

2. Arrange the leaves on a large platter, scatter over the red onion, avocado and the beetroot wedges. Remove the skin and fine bones from the fish, break into large flakes and place the flakes on the salad.

3. Whisk together the dressing ingredients and season to taste with freshly ground black pepper. Dress the salad and toss to coat, scatter over the toasted pumpkin seeds and serve immediately.

Ingredients

2 tablespoons pumpkin seeds
150g baby spinach leaves
100g watercress
½ red onion, thinly sliced
1 avocado, peeled and sliced
2 cooked and peeled beetroot, sliced into wedges
4 fillets smoked mackerel (or peppered, if preferred)

Dressing

3 tablespoons sunflower oil
2 tablespoons balsamic vinegar
1 teaspoon Dijon mustard
Freshly ground black pepper

Per serving: 397 kcals | 25g protein | 31g fat | 10g saturated fat | 9g carbs | 6g sugar | 5g fibre | 2.2g salt

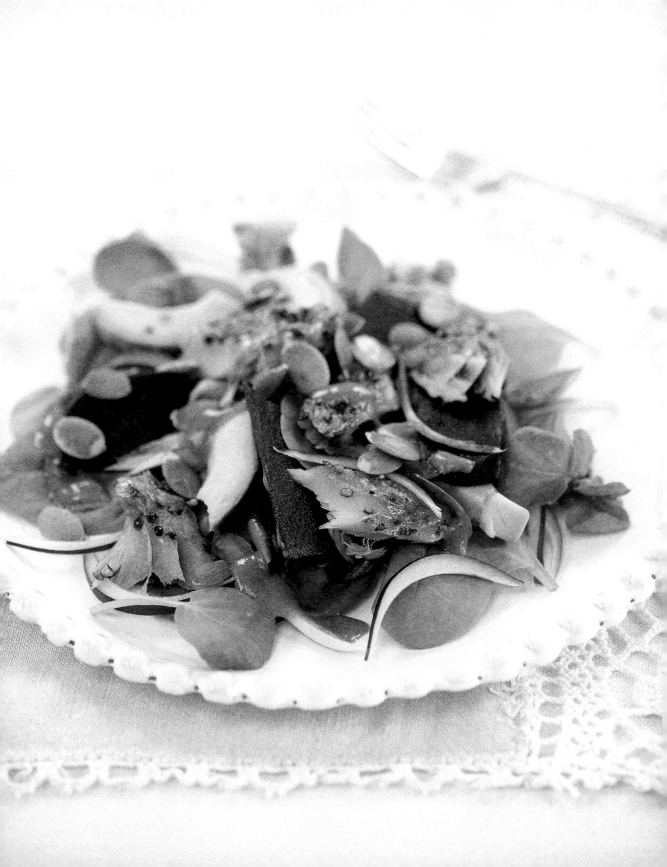

OSTEOPOROSIS

This condition occurs when your bones become weak, fragile and more porous, leading to fractures – most commonly in your spine, wrist and hipbones. After the age of thirty-five, we naturally lose bone density, making it increasingly important to eat plenty of calcium to keep them strong, and avoid foods and drinks that can make them weaker. A diagnosis of osteoporosis is normally made after you fracture a bone, or are identified as being 'high risk'. You will be referred for a bone-density scan, known as a DeXA scan, which will assess how porous your bones are.

THE SCIENCE

Although our bones become more brittle as a natural part of ageing, osteoporosis is a highly preventable disease. Risk factors include having a diet that is poor in calcium and vitamin D, smoking, drinking excessive amounts of alcohol, getting inadequate exercise, being underweight, family history, eating disorders and hormonal imbalance.

Women, in particular, become more prone to osteoporosis as levels of bone-protecting oestrogen dip when their childbearing years draw to an end, and those who have the menopause before forty-five are more at risk. However, men can also suffer from osteoporosis (the risk increases over the age of fifty), and it can be caused by thyroid disorders, diabetes, kidney disease, rheumatoid arthritis, problems with the pancreas, and certain medications, such as high-dose steroids, or any conditions that cause high levels of cortisol (such as Cushing's disease).

At one point, calcium supplementation was regularly suggested for osteoporosis; however, high levels of calcium taken in this way have now been linked to heart disease in men, so it's a better idea to eat a high-calcium diet and get regular, weight-bearing exercise. There are a number of drugs that can help to boost your bone density. For women, HRT can have a protective effect on the bones, but the downsides (such as an increase of cardiovascular disease and breast cancer) can outweigh the benefits.

Foods to Eat

- **Studies have shown that taking calcium and vitamin D supplements** lowers the rate of fractures by thirty-five to fifty per cent, but they must be taken together to avoid cardiovascular problems.

- **Oily fish is not only a good source of vitamin D,** but it also contains essential fats that have been shown to encourage a greater increase in bone formation (see recipe on page 260).

- **A Mediterranean diet** based on fish, fruits and vegetables, whole grains, olive oil and moderate amounts of alcohol, has been shown to benefit bone health.

- **Dairy produce** (such as milk, cheese and yoghurt), leafy green vegetables, almonds, the small bones in tinned salmon or mackerel, sesame and sunflower seeds, and soya are excellent sources of calcium.

- **Plenty of fresh fruit and vegetables,** which contain the minerals potassium and magnesium, can encourage your bones to absorb key minerals, such as calcium. Fruit and vegetables also contain vitamin C and zinc, which are required for bone health.
- **Phytoestrogens,** such as soya, can protect your bones from further loss of density.
- **Vegetable sources of protein,** such as nuts, seeds, tofu and other soya products, and pulses, which can reduce your risk of fractures. Protein helps to build strong bones.

Foods to Avoid

- **More than five servings of red meat a week,** which can increase your risk of fractures.
- **Excessive alcohol** (i.e. binge-drinking) can leach calcium from your bones.
- **Salt and fizzy drinks** cause calcium to be excreted from your body.
- **Excess caffeine** also leaches calcium from bones.
- **Vitamin A supplements** can harm your bones; instead, choose brightly coloured fruit and vegetables, which contain beta-carotene – a natural form of vitamin A, which is much safer.

Expert Tips

- **Make sure you get plenty of natural sunlight,** which is necessary for our bodies to make vitamin D – an essential nutrient for bone health.
- **Smoking is one of the worst things you can do** for bone health, as it leaches calcium directly from your bones. Stop as soon as you can.
- **Get regular, weight-bearing exercise** (such as walking, jogging, tennis, dancing and aerobics) to protect your bones; if you are suffering from osteoporosis, you'll need to see a physiotherapist or specialist trainer to work out a safe programme. Exercise also helps to improve balance, posture and muscle strength, which can help to prevent falls.
- **Maintain a healthy weight** – a low BMI is linked with bone loss in both men and women.
- **Get your thyroid gland checked** regularly.

CASE HISTORY

At sixty-eight, Sylvia was very slim and suffering from pain in her back and ribs. She had experienced quite an early menopause, at forty-three, and used to smoke heavily. She had also been taking thyroxine for years to treat an underactive thyroid (if the dose is too high, this can be a risk factor for osteoporosis). She was a classic case for the onset of osteoporosis, which a bone scan and X-ray confirmed. She increased vitamin D and calcium in her diet, and cut out drinking alcohol and caffeine. She also started a gentle exercise programme, beginning with long walks and swimming, and attended a 'falls' class, which showed her how to prevent accidents that could lead to a fracture. A later scan showed that her bone density had increased slightly; best of all, she was feeling healthier and could advise her daughter of the preventative measures she could take.

WARNING

Ask your GP to arrange a bone-density test if you break a bone over the age of forty-five. Also report any sudden or unexplained change in posture, loss of height or back pain. You may be referred for a DeXA scan if you had an early menopause, if you have a low BMI or if you have taken epilepsy medication long-term.

See also: Menopause, Thyroid problems

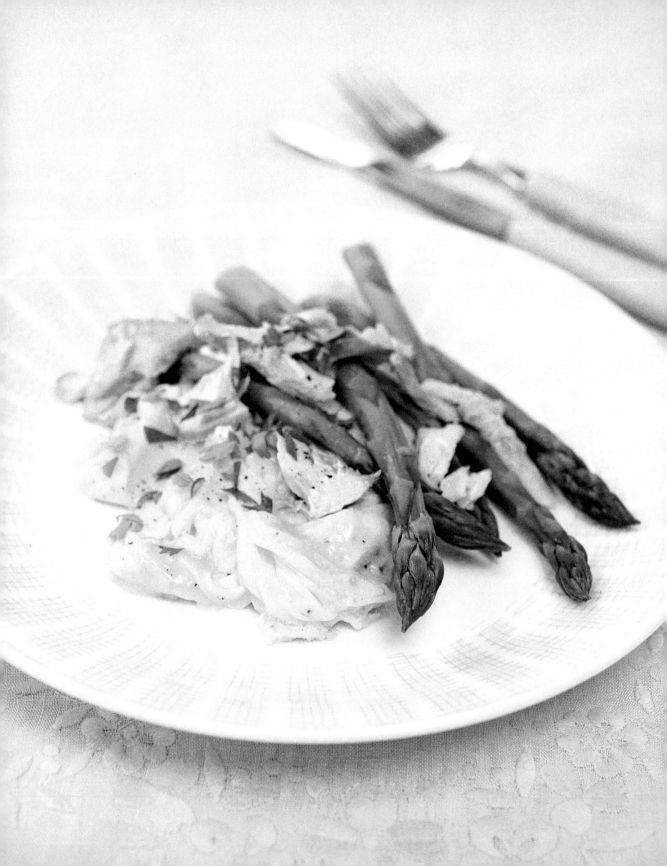

HOT SMOKED SALMON WITH ASPARAGUS AND SCRAMBLED EGGS

Serves 4
Preparation time: 5 minutes
Cooking time: 5 minutes

1. Snap the woody ends off the asparagus and steam the stalks for 4 to 5 minutes until just tender.

2. While the asparagus steams, gently whisk the eggs with the milk and freshly ground black pepper. Heat the butter in a medium non-stick pan until just melted but not browned, pour in the eggs and stir until the eggs are just setting.

3. Divide the eggs between four plates, add the asparagus and break large flakes of the salmon on top, scatter with the parsley and serve immediately.

Ingredients

250g fresh asparagus

8 medium eggs

50ml soya milk (must be calcium enriched) or semi-skimmed milk

Freshly ground black pepper

15g butter

160g hot smoked salmon (or trout if preferred)

2 tablespoons flat leaf parsley, roughly chopped

| Per serving: 324 kcals | 32g protein | 22g fat | 6g saturated fat | 1g carbs | 1g sugar | 1.5g fibre | 2.6g salt |

PARKINSON'S DISEASE

Parkinson's tends to be a disease that elderly people get, but actor Michael J. Fox, diagnosed in his late thirties, is a famous exception to the rule. The first symptoms you might see could be a general slowing down and muscle stiffness. The handwriting of sufferers becomes shaky and they might look depressed because their face muscles flatten out. They may also develop a tremor when their hands are at rest, which improves with movement, and they might walk in a shuffling movement with their feet wide apart. It's a nasty disease because it tends to be progressive.

THE SCIENCE

Parkinson's is caused by a loss of the nerve cells that produce dopamine in the brain, but no one knows why this happens. Dopamine carries messages between the brain and the nervous system and as levels drop, symptoms increase. It is thought there may be a genetic link in Parkinson's and it is also known that exposure to pesticides and the use of street drugs are causes in some cases. There are no conclusive tests to show you have the disease, but evidence based on the weight of symptoms will be taken into account and a SPECT scan or MRI scan may help to confirm the diagnosis.

The only tip for Parkinson's prevention is to avoid taking street drugs. Eating a diet rich in brightly coloured antioxidants (see page 10) will help to reduce oxidative damage to the brain which may contribute to Parkinson's.

The main medication prescribed for Parkinson's, Levodopa (which aims to replace the dopamine in the brain), is difficult for the digestive system to absorb, and protein can reduce its effectiveness, so a special protein redistribution diet may be recommended. On this, you will be advised to eat mainly carb-based meals during the day, and eat most of your protein in the evenings when you are not taking a dose of Levodopa. You should follow the advice of a dietitian on this, and don't decrease the protein you are eating without discussion. A health-care team will be assigned to help you after diagnosis.

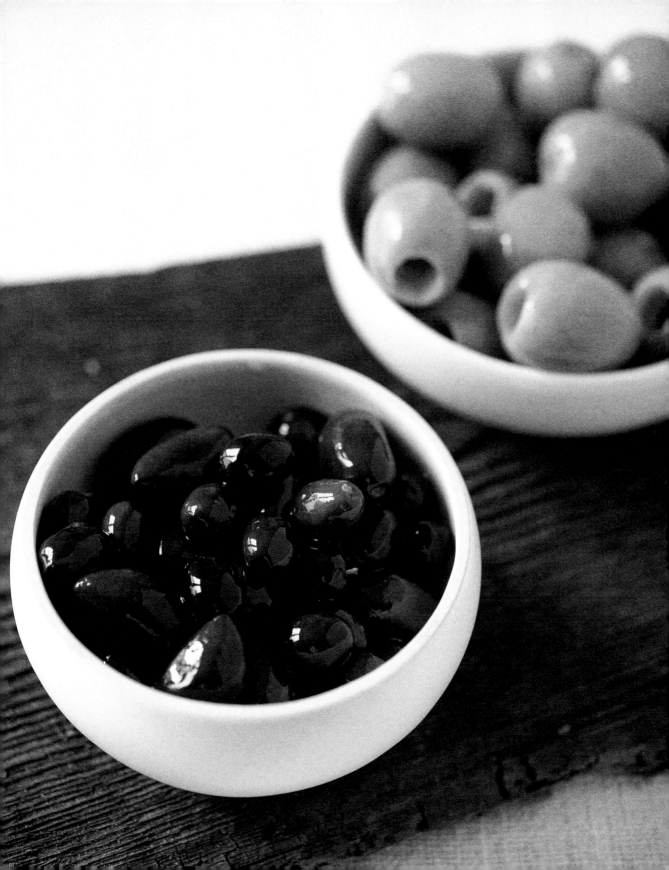

Foods to Eat

- **Follow the dietary advice** of your health-care team to ensure optimum absorption of your medication.

- **Anecdotal evidence suggests that Coenzyme Q10** can slow the progression of Parkinson's disease, but there haven't been clinical trials on this. You could increase your levels of dietary CoQ10, which include organ meats, beef, soya oil, oily fish and peanuts.

- **A high intake of dietary antioxidants** can protect against the development of the disease. Get plenty of vitamin E in particular – from olives, avocados, nuts and fatty fish.

- **Constipation can be a complication of Parkinson's** so plenty of fibre in the diet is essential. Sufferers may have difficulty chewing very fibrous foods, in which case a dietitian will put them on a diet with lots of purees, but as long as you are able, get plenty of whole grains, pulses and vegetables to help your bowels move food along.

- **Drink two litres of fluid a day.** Plain water is best, but you can also have fruit and vegetable juices and smoothies, and tea in moderation.

Expert Tips

- **Antacid indigestion remedies can interfere** with the absorption of drugs, so don't take them at the same time as Parkinson's medication.

- **Get in touch with Parkinson's UK** for loads of advice and support: www.parkinsons.org.uk.

- **Read Michael J. Fox's autobiography** *Lucky Me* for an uplifting story of how one sufferer has coped with the disease.

- **There is some evidence that coffee drinkers** have a reduced risk of developing Parkinson's.

CASE STUDY

Alex was a sixty-five-year-old retired schoolteacher who painted watercolours as a hobby. His friends noticed that he seemed to be slowing down in his movements and worried that he looked depressed, but the first symptom Alex noticed was that he wasn't able to make the clean brushstrokes that he used to when painting. When he signed his name, it didn't look quite right. His friends eventually suggested that he visit his doctor and after a neurological examination, he was diagnosed with Parkinson's. He started taking some medications, which helped with the symptoms, and joined a support group, which he found helped him to adjust. He also modified his diet to include more fibre and antioxidants, and two years after diagnosis, he is still enjoying painting.

See also: Constipation, Depression, Dementia, Insomnia, Restless Legs

PROSTATE PROBLEMS

In young men, the prostate gland is about the size of a walnut, but it tends to enlarge as they get older. Over the age of fifty-five, men may find they have symptoms of an enlarged prostate, such as not being able to hold their urine, having to get up frequently in the night to urinate, and having trouble urinating when they get to the loo, with only a dribble coming out. If you experience these symptoms, you should consult a doctor because they can be warning signs of prostate cancer – but equally they could just be caused by the enlargement of the prostate. Some types of prostate cancer are aggressive and spread quickly to the rest of the body, but most aren't. It's said that most men die with prostate cancer rather than because of it. But don't let that stop you having any symptoms checked as soon as you notice them, just in case.

THE SCIENCE

An enlarged prostate gland pressing on the urethra is often what causes changes in urination in older men. Known as benign prostatic hyperplasia (BPH commonly), this is a treatable condition, so do consult your doctor.

Prostate cancer is more common in white and Afro-Caribbean men than in South-east Asians. It seems to run in families, and you will be more susceptible if you are overweight, don't take regular exercise and eat an unhealthy diet. Rates of prostate cancer appear to be lower in men who eat a lot of foods containing lycopene (tomatoes and red fruits) and selenium (the best source is Brazil nuts), so it may be worth increasing the quantities of these in your diet.

Sometimes doctors will decide not to treat prostate cancer, depending on the type and size of the tumour, because it may not present a risk of spreading. Men with cancers more likely to spread may have to undergo surgery, chemotherapy or radiotherapy, and there is a risk that this could affect their sex life afterwards, and possibly cause incontinence. We say this only to urge you to get any symptoms checked out early. Men are notoriously bad at consulting their GP about subjects of a delicate nature like this, but isn't it worth a quick rectal examination if it will mean you can continue to have a healthy sex life into old age? We think so!

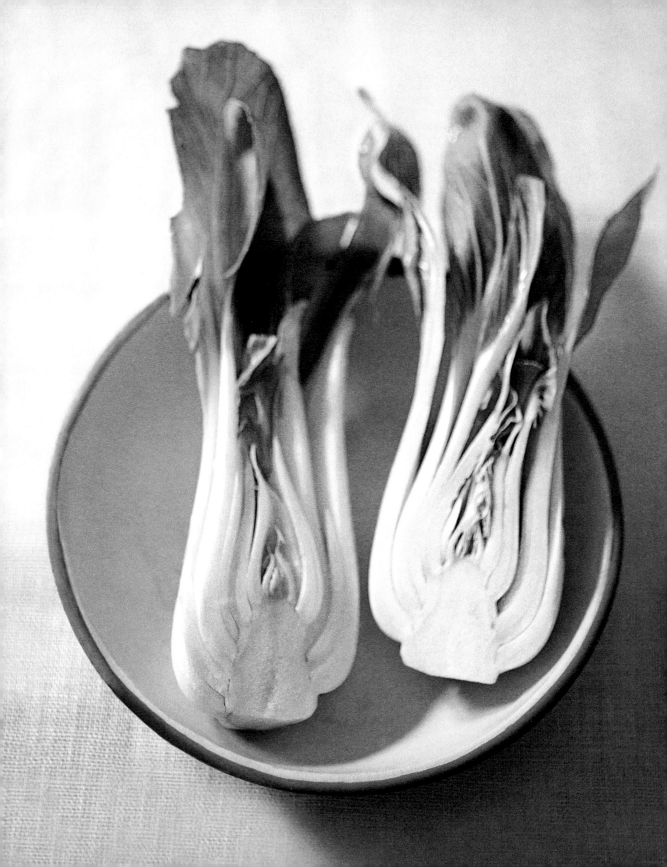

Foods to Eat

- There's evidence that the Mediterranean diet may help to protect against prostate cancer. Lycopene, found in tomatoes, may be an important antioxidant for prostate health, although there is also evidence to the contrary! The other main ingredients of the diet – olives and olive oil, fish, whole grains, and red wine in moderation drunk with meals – are all associated with living longer and reducing your risk of cardiovascular disease and cancer.

- There's lots of evidence that a diet rich in vegetables reduces the risk of prostate cancer. Aim for well over five portions a day.

- There's also anecdotal evidence that plant sterols, found in cholesterol-lowering yoghurts and spreads, can reduce the size of the prostate.

- Eat more Asian-style foods, such as soy products, rice, and green and yellow vegetables (broccoli, pak choi and kohlrabi are good).

- Zinc is important for prostate health. Get it from seafood, whole grains, pumpkin seeds and pulses.

- A diet high in fibre may help to flush out male hormones in the gut and reduce prostate enlargement.

Foods to Avoid

- Keep saturated (animal) fats to a minimum. If you must have red meat, cut the visible fat off before cooking and avoid processed meats such as sausages and burgers.

- Caffeine and alcohol are diuretics that could make you need to get up and urinate more often in the night.

Expert Tips

- Getting regular exercise and maintaining a healthy weight will offer protection against prostate cancer.

- Saw palmetto is a remedy that's said to improve urinary flow and shrink an enlarged prostate, although there's no substantial evidence of this.

- For more advice, see the website www.prostate-cancer.org.uk/toolkits/diet-and-prostate-cancer.

CASE STUDY

Sixty-six-year-old year old Ian was embarrassed at how often he had to go to the loo during the chess matches he enjoyed playing with friends. After getting to the urinal, nothing would happen for a long time until he finally passed a dribble of urine. This experience repeated itself an hour later. He also was finding that he was tired in the morning because he had to get up three or four times a night to urinate. He went to his doctor, who gave him a rectal examination and diagnosed an enlarged prostate. Some further tests followed, along with a trial of medication, which helped. His doctor encouraged him to take up some more active hobbies and he joined a walking club. He also took Ian off the diuretic blood pressure medication he was on and prescribed an alternative one. Ian switched to decaf coffee and tea and monitored how much he drank in the evenings, and his urinary symptoms are much more controlled.

See also: Cancer, High cholesterol

CHILLI CON CARNE WITH LENTILS

Serves 4
Preparation time: 5 minutes
Cooking time: 1 hour

1. Heat the oil in a large saucepan or casserole dish over a medium heat, add the onion, cover and cook for 5 minutes or until soft and translucent but not coloured. Break the mince up with your fingers and add to the pan, turn the heat up a little and brown for 5 minutes, stirring frequently. Add the garlic and carrots and continue to cook for 1 minute, seasoning with a little salt and freshly ground black pepper.

2. Add the spices to the pan and stir for a minute before adding the tinned tomatoes and purée. Bring to a simmer, put a lid on and continue to simmer for 40 minutes. You may want to give it a stir after 20 minutes.

3. Add the kidney beans, lentils and chocolate to the pan and simmer for a further 10 minutes, then stir in the fresh tomatoes and warm though for 1 minute.

4. Serve with the cooked brown rice.

Ingredients

1 tablespoon sunflower oil
1 onion, finely chopped
300g lean beef mince
2 cloves garlic, crushed
2 carrots, peeled and grated coarsely
Sea salt and freshly ground black pepper
½ teaspoon dried chilli flakes
½ teaspoon hot chilli powder
1 teaspoon smoked paprika
1 teaspoon ground cumin
1 teaspoon dried oregano
2 x 400g tins chopped tomatoes
3 tablespoons tomato puree
1 x 400g tin kidney beans, rinsed and drained
1 x 400g tin lentils, rinsed and drained
1 cube dark chocolate
4 tomatoes, roughly chopped

To Serve

Cooked brown rice

| Per serving: 387 kcals | 30g protein | 12.5g fat | 4.5g saturated fat | 41g carbs | 18g sugar | 14g fibre | 1.1g salt |

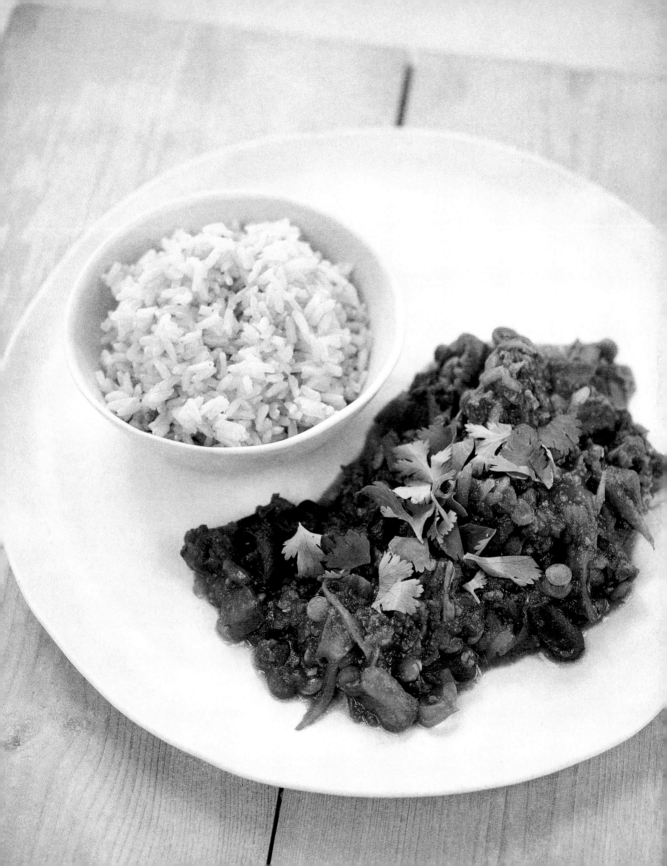

STROKE

The sooner you get help for someone suffering a stroke, the better their chances of making a full recovery. The acronym FAST was coined to help the public recognize the symptoms, which are not always obvious. F stands for facial weakness: can the person smile or is their Face drooping on one or both sides? Can they raise both Arms? Can they Speak clearly, or do their words sound muffled or slurred? If the answer to any of these questions is no, then it's Time to call for an ambulance.

THE SCIENCE

Ninety per cent of strokes are ischaemic strokes, in which blood vessels become blocked, cutting off the blood supply to part of the brain. The blockage can be caused by arteries getting clogged up with plaque or by a blood clot that has travelled from somewhere else (as in cardiovascular disease). The remaining ten per cent of strokes are haemorrhagic, caused when an artery ruptures and bleeds into the brain. Transient ischaemic attacks (TIAs) are so-called 'mini strokes'. The symptoms might last just a few minutes and always resolve within twenty-four hours, after which the sufferer feels perfectly well again, but they are a warning sign: once you've had a TIA you are at increased risk of getting other, more significant strokes. If you experience any kind of visual disturbance, dizziness, nausea or loss of balance for no obvious reason, consult your doctor because it may have been a mini-stroke. Don't take it lightly, no matter what your age, because you might need treatment to reduce the risk of a recurrence.

Measures for prevention of strokes are the same as for cardiovascular disease: don't smoke, don't drink excessive amounts of alcohol, keep yourself at a healthy weight, exercise regularly, keep your blood pressure and blood cholesterol at healthy levels, take steps to deal with any stress in your life, and eat a balanced, varied diet full of fresh fruit and vegetables, whole grains and healthy oils.

If a close relative has had a stroke, your risk is higher; if you are South Asian or Afro-Caribbean you are also more likely to have a stroke, because these groups have more risk of high blood pressure and/or high cholesterol; diabetics have a higher risk; and being over the age of sixty-five makes you more at risk – although a quarter of strokes every year happen to people younger than this. Being in an at-risk group makes it even more important that you take preventative measures.

If someone has a stroke, the first twenty-four hours are crucial in determining how much brain function will be affected. Aggressive physiotherapy in the following three months can definitely improve the outcome. But, basically, a stroke is not good news and you are well advised to take whatever steps you can to avoid it.

If you have high cholesterol levels, you may be advised to follow the Portfolio Diet (see page 244). For high blood pressure, the DASH diet is very effective (see page 240). Otherwise, for general stroke prevention follow a Mediterranean-style diet with lots of olive oil, garlic, tomatoes, onions, fresh fish, whole grains, multi-coloured fruits and vegetables, and perhaps a glass of red wine with the evening meal.

Folic acid and vitamin B12 supplements may be recommended by your consultant.

Eat plenty of omega-3-containing foods: oily fish, olive oil, nuts and seeds.

Saturated fats found in animal foods and shop-bought cakes, biscuits, pastries and ready meals will increase your risk of stroke.

Salt should be kept to a minimum, by reading labels on any packaged food and cooking from fresh whenever you can.

Heavy drinking trebles your risk of having a stroke, because it raises blood pressure and causes atrial fibrillation (an irregular heartbeat – see below).

Atrial fibrillation, where the heart beats irregularly, is a risk factor for stroke. If you ever get palpitations, breathlessness or chest pain, or if your pulse feels irregular over the course of a minute, then consult your GP, who can refer you for tests.

As with cardiovascular disease, cocaine use can cause strokes in young people, and you don't need to be a habitual user; it could just as easily happen the first time you try it.

It's never too late to start getting regular exercise but if you haven't donned trainers since your school days and that's a while ago now, join a gym and get a trainer to work out a programme for you rather than launching straight into training for a marathon.

You'll find useful advice on the Stroke Association website: www.stroke.org.uk.

WARNING

Always consult a doctor about any symptoms that could indicate you have had a TIA (see above). You should also get immediate help if you experience a severe, sudden-onset headache, as this could indicate a haemorrhagic stroke. And always call an ambulance if someone loses consciousness for no obvious reason and doesn't come round straight away.

See also: Cardiovascular disease, High blood pressure, High cholesterol

THYROID PROBLEMS

The thyroid gland is basically the body's accelerator pedal. It secretes a hormone called thyroxine that sets the speed at which your metabolism and body systems work. So if your thyroid is underactive, you feel slow, lethargic and tired; if it is overactive, you are over-cranked.

Thyroid problems are more common in women. If you are thinking to yourself that it might be a good thing to have an overactive thyroid, think again, because if you are producing too much thyroxine you will burn out pretty quickly. And if you have too little thyroxine, some body systems might start to break down, so your heart rate could become too slow (or too fast), and your digestive system could become sluggish. Each condition is dangerous and needs appropriate medical treatment.

THE SCIENCE

Thyroxine is one of the few hormones in the body that is dependent on one particular element in the diet, and that element is iodine. If your diet is low in iodine or if you don't absorb it efficiently for some reason, you won't produce enough thyroxine. Most dietary iodine comes from milk, but there is increasing evidence that levels in the UK population are not as high as they used to be. Your thyroid gland will still be stimulated to produce it but won't be able to, and the gland will swell, causing a thick lump in the neck that we call a goiter. Occasionally, if it's left untreated, this can develop into a cancerous tumour.

There's a particular type of thyroid disease called Graves disease, which is an autoimmune problem. It starts with an overproduction of thyroxine, but sufferers can end up with an underactive thyroid. People with this condition can get swollen, stary eyes. If you can see the whites of the eyes above the pupil, this may be a sign of an overactive thyroid. Hashimoto's thyroiditis is an auto-immune condition where the thyroid tends to become underactive.

If you are over-producing thyroxine, you can take medication to reduce it, but there are occasionally toxic side effects, so you can't stay on it for life. The next step would be surgery to remove part of the gland, or you might be given radioactive iodine, which kills off the thyroxine-producing cells.

Foods to Eat

- **To prevent thyroid problems,** you need adequate iodine in the diet. Good sources include sea vegetables, such as kelp, fish and seafood (see recipe on page 275). Cereals and vegetables grown in areas with a high iodine content in the soil are also useful, but you'd have to ask a local farmer to find out because they don't tend to mention this on the packaging!

- **Tyrosine, an amino acid found in** red meat, fish and dairy products, almonds, avocado, banana, seeds, lima beans, wheat and oats, is needed to produce thyroxine.

- **Eat adequate vitamin A** (from organ meats, and yellowy-orange vegetables such as carrots and pumpkins) and vitamin D (from liver, eggs and oily fish), and make sure you get enough exposure to sunlight.

- **If you have an overactive thyroid,** eat plenty of Brussels sprouts, cabbage, spinach, cauliflower, kale and soya products, as there's evidence that they can suppress thyroxine production. On the same note, avoid them if you have an underactive thyroid.

Foods to Avoid

- **If your thyroid is over-active,** the last thing you need is anything that speeds up the metabolism, so avoid caffeine in all its forms (tea, coffee, cola, and painkilling drugs). Alcohol intake should also be severely limited.

CASE STUDY

Jeanine was a forty-year-old, stick-thin gym addict. She ate lots and did muscle-building exercise but still couldn't put on weight. She considered herself a 'high-stress' individual, prone to anxiety, and her relationships at work were often strained because of this. She sweated even when she wasn't doing anything, and had a fine tremor that she was self-conscious about. She didn't think it was worth going to see her doctor until she noticed that she was having discomfort swallowing. Her doctor noted a swelling in the neck, and blood tests revealed an over-active thyroid. Jeanine started taking meds to control the tremor and after a few months underwent treatment to disable the over-active thyroid. Soon she gained weight and got up to a healthy BMI, and felt much more relaxed. She couldn't believe the stress she'd experienced for so long had been due to a treatable condition!

WARNING

Some cancers can also cause an overactive thyroid, so make sure you get checked out by your GP.

See also: Constipation, High blood pressure, Low sex drive

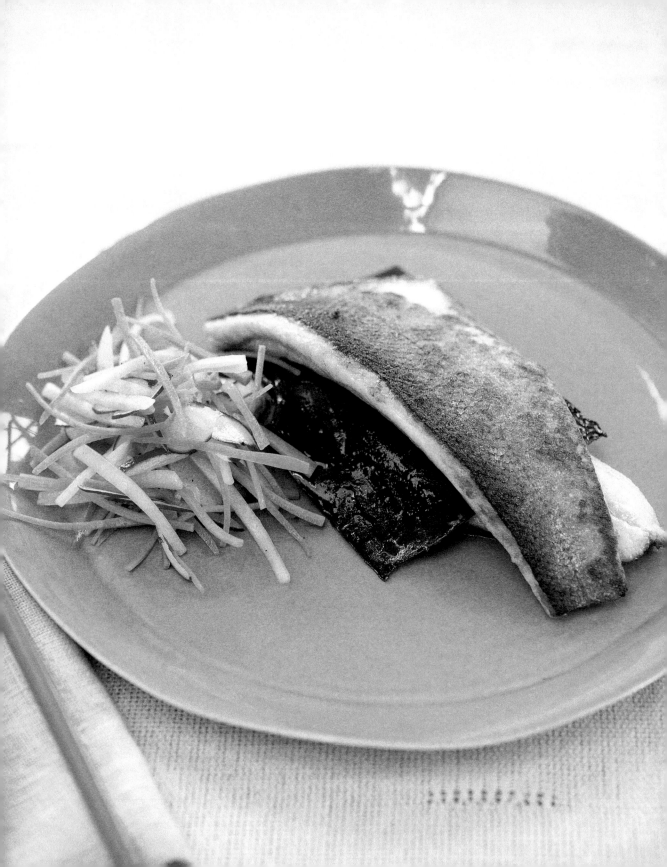

PAN-FRIED KELP SEA BASS WITH CUCUMBER, DAIKON AND CARROT SALAD

Serves 4
Preparation time: 25 minutes
Cooking time: 6 minutes

1. Place the dried kombu on a large plate and gently rub the sake into its leathery leaves. Leave to soften for 10 minutes.

2. Sandwich the kombu between the two fillets of each fish. Rub the olive oil on to the skin of the fish. Set aside for 15 minutes.

3. In a large bowl, whisk together the vinegar, oil, mustard seeds and sugar, season with freshly ground pepper. Add the cucumber, daikon and carrot to the dressing and toss to coat the vegetables.

4. Heat a large frying pan over a medium-high heat, discard the kombu and fry the fish skin side down for 2 to 3 minutes, turn over and cook for a further 2 to 3 minutes. Serve immediately with the salad.

Ingredients

For the Fish

4 x 10cm pieces dried kombu (kelp)

1 tablespoon sake or mirin

4 x 450g sea bass, filleted (you can use frozen seabass fillets, but make sure they are fully defrosted before using)

1 tablespoon extra-virgin olive oil

For the Salad

2 tablespoons rice wine vinegar

1 tablespoon extra-virgin olive oil

1 teaspoon yellow mustard seeds

Pinch of caster sugar

Freshly ground black pepper

½ cucumber, peeled, halved and thinly sliced

150g radishes or daikon, peeled and finely shredded

2 carrots, peeled and thinly sliced

| Per serving: 491 kcals | 78g protein | 16g fat | 2.5g saturated fat | 8g carbs | 7g sugar | 3.5g fibre | 0.8g salt |

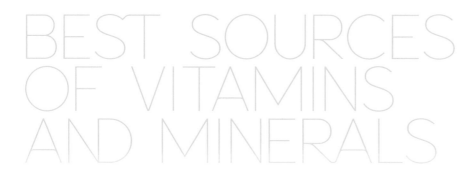

BEST SOURCES OF VITAMINS AND MINERALS

VITAMINS

A: Retinol in animal foods and beta-carotene in plant foods.

Beta-carotene: brightly coloured fruits and vegetables, including apricots, carrots, leafy green vegetables, squash and melon.

Retinol: Liver, oily fish, eggs, butter and cheese.

B1 (thiamine): Asparagus, mushrooms, spinach, sunflower seeds, tuna, pulses, tomatoes, aubergine, whole grains.

B2 (Riboflavin): Asparagus, chard, broccoli, venison, eggs, yoghurt, cows' milk, liver, spinach.

B3 (Niacin): Pulses, mushrooms, liver, halibut, asparagus, venison, chicken, salmon, sea vegetables, tuna, sardines, Romaine lettuce.

B5 (Pantothenic Acid): Mushrooms, cauliflower, sunflower seeds, sweetcorn, yoghurt, broccoli.

B6 (Pyridoxine): Spinach, peppers, cauliflower, bananas, celery, asparagus, broccoli, cod, kale, garlic, tuna, cabbage, Brussels sprouts, Marmite.

B12 (Cyanocobalamin): Organ meats, sardines, snapper, venison, scallops, beef, lamb, yoghurt, cow's milk, eggs.

Biotin: Romaine lettuce, carrots, almonds, eggs, onions, cabbage, cucumber, cauliflower, milk, raspberries, strawberries, halibut, oats, walnuts.

Folic Acid: Romaine lettuce, spinach, asparagus, liver, parsley, broccoli, cauliflower, beets, pulses.

C (Ascorbic acid): Fresh fruit and vegetables, particularly broccoli, peppers, kale, cauliflower, berries, lemons and limes, kiwi, papaya, cabbage, citrus fruit, tomatoes, courgettes, asparagus, celery, pineapples, lettuce, melon, peppermint, parsley.

D (calciferols): Milk products, eggs, oily fish, fish oil. Synthesized in the skin from sunlight.

E (tocopherols): Nuts, seeds, eggs, milk, whole grains, unrefined oils, leafy vegetables, avocados, soya, kiwi, tomatoes, blueberries, papaya, parsley.

K: Molasses, spinach, Brussels sprouts, green beans, asparagus, broccoli, kale, green peas, carrots, cod liver oil, cabbage, avocados. Synthesized in the intestines.

MINERALS

Calcium: Leafy green vegetables, molasses, yoghurt (and other dairy produce), sesame seeds, almonds, green beans, garlic, oranges, asparagus, celery, broccoli.

Chromium: Whole grains, onions, tomatoes, brewer's yeast, oysters, liver, potatoes.

Copper: Liver, molasses, chard, spinach, sesame seeds, kale, courgettes, asparagus, aubergine, cashews, tomatoes, green beans, ginger, potatoes.

Iodine: Sea vegetables, yoghurt, milk, eggs, strawberries, some fish and shellfish.

Iron: Chard, spinach, turmeric, Romaine lettuce, molasses, tofu, green beans, beef (and other red meats), poultry, asparagus, broccoli, leeks, kelp, dried fruit (in particular apricots).

Magnesium: Spinach, chard, courgettes, broccoli, halibut, pumpkin seeds, cucumber, green beans, sesame seeds, sunflower seeds, flaxseeds, celery, kale.

Manganese: Kale, chard, raspberries, pineapple, Romaine lettuce, spinach, maple syrup, molasses, garlic, grapes, courgettes, strawberries, oats, spelt, green beans, brown rice, leeks, tofu, broccoli, beets, whole wheat.

Phosphorus: Tuna, mackerel, sardines, salmon, anchovies, trout, liver, turkey, chicken, eggs, pine nuts, pistachios, pumpkin seeds, sesame seeds, walnuts, almonds, brazil nuts, cashews, soya, cheese, whole grains, chocolate.

Potassium: Chard, spinach, fennel, kale, Brussels sprouts, broccoli, butternut squash, acorn squash, molasses, aubergine, cantaloupe melon, tomatoes, cucumber, peppers, apricots, ginger, strawberries, avocado, tuna, cabbage.

Selenium: Brazil nuts, mushrooms, cod, prawns, tuna, snapper, halibut, liver, salmon, turkey, sardines.

Sodium: Salt; found in processed foods of all kinds.

Zinc: Sea vegetables, spinach, pumpkin seeds, yeast, beef, lamb, liver, mushrooms, spinach, courgettes, asparagus, chard, miso, maple syrup, broccoli, peas, yoghurt, pumpkin seeds, sesame seeds.

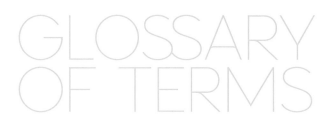

GLOSSARY OF TERMS

ADHD (attention deficit hyperactivity syndrome): see page 108.

AMD (age-related macular degeneration): see page 106.

Amino acid: The basic building blocks of proteins; there are twenty altogether – eleven of which can be synthesized by the body, and another nine that you must get from the protein in your diet.

Antioxidant: Nutrients, found mainly in fresh fruit and vegetables, that protect your body from 'free radicals', which cause the degenerative processes of ageing. Some examples of antioxidants include beta-carotene, vitamins A, C and E, lutein, lycopene and quercetin (see pages 11–13).

Aspartame: An artificial sweetener (which contains a source of phenylalanine) used in low-calorie products.

Auto-immune disease: A health condition caused by an overactive immune response by your body against its own tissues. In other words, your body attacks its own cells. Rheumatoid arthritis is an example of an auto-immune condition.

Beta-carotene/carotenoids: Beta-carotene is a 'carotenoid' that is found in colourful fruits and vegetables. It is a 'precursor' to vitamin A, which means that the body uses this nutrient to make vitamin A.

Bioavailable: A term indicating how easily a substance is absorbed into your bloodstream and used by your body. Some foods contain vitamins and minerals that are more bioavailable than others.

Biopsy: An examination of tissues removed from your body to establish the type, presence or cause of a disease. You may have a biopsy of your intestines, for example, to check your colon health.

BMI (body mass index): A measurement based on your height and weight, which gives an estimate of your body fat. It is used to find out if you are under-, over- or normal weight, or obese (see page 59).

BPH (benign prostatic hyperplasia): see page 265.

CFS (chronic fatigue syndrome): see page 114.

Cholesterol: A waxy substance found in the body that is needed to produce hormones, vitamin D and bile (which is required for digestion). Low-density lipoprotein (LDL) cholesterol is considered to be 'bad' cholesterol because elevated LDL levels are associated with an increased risk of cardiovascular disease. High-density lipoprotein (HDL) cholesterol is known as 'good' cholesterol, as it is associated with lower levels of cardiovascular disease.

Colonoscopy: An examination of the inside of your colon and rectum, which your doctor will undertake by using a flexible tube (known as a colonoscope) with a camera on the end.

Cortisol: A hormone released by the adrenal glands when we are stressed. It increases blood pressure and blood sugar levels, and suppresses the immune system

CT scan: A computed tomography (CT) scan is a type of scan that uses x-rays to create cross-sectional pictures of your body.

CVD (cardiovascular disease): see page 228.

DeXA (Dual energy X-ray absorptiometry) scan: An imaging test that measures bone density (the amount of bone mineral contained in a certain volume of bone) by passing x-rays with two different energy levels through the bone. It is used to diagnose osteoporosis (see page 258).

Dopamine: A neurotransmitter (chemical messenger) in the brain, which is essential for the healthy functioning of your central nervous system (and emotional health).

EFAs (Essential fatty acids): Otherwise known as 'omega oils' (3, 6 and 9; see page 16), found mainly in nuts, seeds, plants and oily fish, which are essential for the smooth functioning of your body and optimum health.

Endorphins: A group of hormones that are secreted in your brain and nervous system, which have a number of functions in your body, including reducing pain, lifting mood and relaxing your mind and body.

Endoscopy: Examination of 'hollow' organs (such as the throat or stomach) with a lighted instrument (called an endoscope), often with a camera on the end.

Flavinols/flavonoids: Plant pigments (colours, such as anthocyanins) that are beneficial to health. Flavonoids have antioxidant, anti-inflammatory and anti-viral properties, among other things. Flavinols are a special class of antioxidants (found in chocolate, for example) that can increase blood flow to brain and heart.

Free radical: The by-product of damage to the cells of the body, from smoking, pollution, poison, unhealthy foods and natural metabolic pathways. This damage is associated with many chronic diseases. Antioxidants can reduce the damage (see page 11).

GI (Glycaemic Index): Which measures the effects of carbohydrates on blood sugar levels (see page 14).

GL (Glycaemic Load): Takes into account the Glycaemic Index rating of a food as well as the protein size to give the most accurate way of predicting how foods affect our blood sugar.

HIV (human immuno-deficiency virus): see page 248.

HRT (hormone replacement therapy): see page 150.

Hydrogenated fats: Also known as 'trans fats', these are manufactured fats created by 'hydrogenation', a process that makes oils solid at room temperature. Associated with heart disease and other health problems.

IBS (irritable bowel syndrome): see page 54.

Insulin resistance: A condition in which the body has a reduced response to the hormone insulin, which is necessary to stabilize blood sugar levels (see page 232).

IUD (Intra-uterine device [coil]): A device used for birth control.

Ketosis: A condition that occurs when the body begins to use fat stores for energy. It can be dangerous.

Laparoscopy: A surgical procedure in which a laparascope (instrument with a light and camera at the end) is inserted through the abdominal wall to view organs or guide surgery.

Lycopene: A red, antioxidant pigment that is present in many fruits, such as tomatoes.

ME (myalgic encephalomyelitis): see page 114.

Micronutrient: A substance, such as vitamins and minerals, which is essential in tiny amounts for health.

Monounsaturated fats: Healthy fats found in olive oil, avocados, almonds, peanuts and sunflower oil. They may lower our risk of heart disease and stroke.

MRI (Magnetic resonance imaging) scan: A type of scan that uses magnetic waves to create pictures of an area of your body.

MS (multiple sclerosis): see page 254.

MSG (Monosodium glutamate): is a food additive used to enhance flavour. Found in many processed foods, and Chinese food in particular.

Neurotransmitters: Chemical messengers that are released from the end of nerve fibres and then transferred to another fibre to provide information (nerve impulses) that travel throughout the body.

Nitrates: A chemical that is found naturally in some foods, such as lettuce and spinach (and water) and used as a preservative in others (such as preserved meats). As a preservative, it is linked with health problems.

NSAIDs (non-steroidal anti-inflammatories): Drugs such as ibuprofen or indomethacin used for their anti-inflammatory and painkilling qualities.

Omega oils/fatty acids: Essential fatty acids that are numbered 3, 6 and 9. Omega oils are a type of unsaturated fat found in fish and plants (including seeds and many nuts) that are known to be beneficial to health.

Pathogen: A bacteria, fungus, parasite, virus or any other micro-organism that can cause disease.

PCBs: Environmental pollutants that are linked with health problems.

PCOS (Polycystic Ovary Syndrome): see page 154.

pH (potential of Hydrogen): The balance of acid and alkaline levels in a solution.

Phytoestrogen: Naturally occurring 'plant oestrogens' that can either increase oestrogen in the body or reduce it.

Phytonutrient: Nutrients (such as beta-carotene), which occur naturally in plants.

PMS (pre-menstrual syndrome): see page 158.

Polyphenol: A group of nutrients that have health benefits; found in many fruits, vegetables and other plants, they are classified as antioxidants.

Polyunsaturated fats: A type of fat that can reduce the risk of cancer, arthritis, diabetes and high cholesterol; high in omega oils, they are found in flaxseeds, sunflower and corn oils.

Probiotics: Healthy, live micro-organisms (usually bacteria) that are similar to the healthy bacteria (flora) found in the gut; probiotics stimulate the growth of flora to achieve good intestinal health.

Pro-oxidant: A substance that can cause oxidative stress (free radicals; see page 10), which is linked with ill health and ageing.

RLS (restless leg syndrome): see page 208.

Saturated fats: Fats that usually occur in animal foods, such as meat and dairy produce; high levels are associated with health problems, such as heart disease. They also occur in palm and coconut oils.

Serotonin: A chemical released in the brain, which regulates sleep, mood, learning and the constriction of the blood vessels.

Sigmoidoscopy: A test that looks inside your rectum via a flexible tube, to assess the health of the lower third of your colon.

SPECT (Single photon emission computed tomography) scan: A type of scan that uses gamma rays to provide a 3D image of your organs, to assess how well they are working.

STD/STI: Sexually transmitted diseases (or sexually transmitted infections), such as Chlamydia.

Sulphites: Food preservatives (E numbers 220 to 228) that can cause health problems (such as breathing difficulties) in some people.

TIA (transient ischaemic attack): see page 270.

Transfats: The common name for hydrogenated fats (see page 16) that are associated with health problems.

Unit of alcohol: In the UK, one unit is 10ml of pure alcohol. This is equivalent to half a pint of beer that has the strength of 3.5 per cent. A 175ml glass of wine with a strength of 12 per cent is two units. A 25ml measure of spirits is one unit. There's a good unit calculator at www.drinkaware. co.uk.

UV rays: Ultraviolet rays are invisible solar radiation rays found in sunlight.

WHR (waist-to-hip ratio): The ratio of the circumference of your waist to that of your hips. It's used to determine your risk of heart disease and other serious health conditions (see page 60).

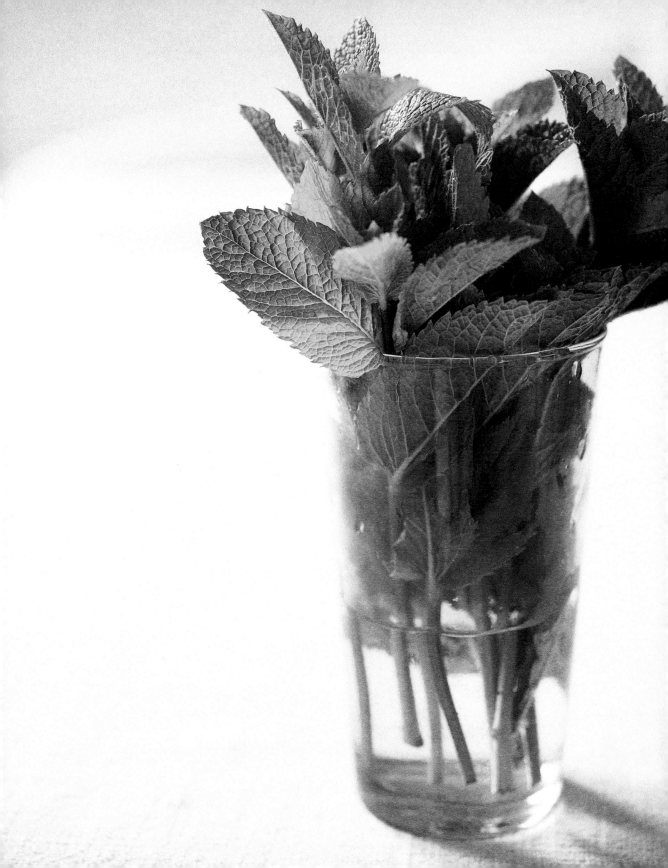

INDEX

ACKNOWLEDGEMENTS

Penguin would like to thank all the brilliant people who have contributed to the making of *The Food Hospital*.

A huge thank you to Gill Paul, who helped with the creation of the text. Thank you to Susan Bell for her gorgeous photography and to Louisa Carter and Annie Hudson for the delicious food. Thank you also to Jo Harris for her beautiful styling.

From Penguin, thank you to Laura Herring, John Hamilton, Sarah Fraser, James Blackman, Nick Lowndes, Anna Derkacz, Jo Wickham, Francesca Russell, Ruth Spencer, Rebecca Blackstone and Gail Jones.

Thank you to everyone at Betty, particularly Liz Warner, Walter Iuzzolino, Sarah Freethy, Lisette Black, Lorne Townend, Brad Evans, Neil Smith, Sophy Walker, Beth Heald and Dr George Grimble. And, of course, a massive thank you to Dr Gio Miletto, Dr Shaw Somers and Lucy Jones.

From Channel Four, thank you to Tanya Shaw. And also a big thank you to Rowan Lawton at PFD.